Everything You Hoped You'd Never Need to Know About Colorectal Cancer

Everything You Hoped You'd Never Need to Know About Colorectal Cancer

DR ANISHA PATEL

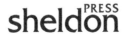

First published in Great Britain by Sheldon Press in 2023
An imprint of John Murray Press
A division of Hodder & Stoughton Ltd,
An Hachette UK company

1

A CIP catalogue record for this title is available from the British Library

Trade Paperback ISBN 9781399811132
eBook ISBN 9781399811170

Typeset by KnowledgeWorks Global Ltd.

Printed and bound in Great Britain by Clays Ltd, Elcograf S.p.A.

John Murray Press policy is to use papers that are natural, renewable and recyclable
products and made from wood grown in sustainable forests. The logging and
manufacturing processes are expected to conform to the environmental regulations
of the country of origin.

John Murray Press
Carmelite House
50 Victoria Embankment
London EC4Y 0DZ

www.sheldonpress.co.uk

To my surgical and medical teams, the countless therapists I visited, the online community, my family and friends, my husband and my gorgeous children – without you there would be no hope. You have been my unbreakable shield. You are my constant. It is you who have carried me to this place I stand today.

And from the bottom of my heart, I sincerely thank you for your lifeline.

Acknowledgements

First and foremost, I would like to thank my incredible children, Kiran and Shani, from the bottom of my heart, and remind them just how much I love them. Without them, this book would likely remain just a pipe dream, an item on my bucket list, a figment of my imagination, as it was they who both encouraged and cajoled me to put pen to paper when I was offered the opportunity to write. Your belief in me gave me the confidence to take that leap of faith. As you both promised, you never once begrudged me the time that I have invested in writing this book, which highlights how very much you wanted me to take on this challenge. And as much as I am so very proud of you, with all that you've been through, all that you do and all that you achieve, I hope this book makes you feel proud of me too.

To my fabulous family, friends, my family friends, and my dream team, my forever friends, my lifelong family friends, my Lovely Ladies, and my Spice girls. I'm so fortunate to have too many of you to name individually but you know who you are and I love you all. I can't even begin to express how much the love and support you have shown my family and I since my diagnosis and beyond, has helped me in getting through treatment, and then learning to deal with the aftermath. Your unwavering support, through all my crazy antics, climbing aboard the rollercoaster that no one ever really wanted to experience, humouring my every suggestion, and listening to my every whim. Thank you for believing in me and giving me the confidence to go forth, for supporting me wherever life takes me, and for embracing with me the spontaneity that life can so richly offer.

To Victoria, my editor – we got there! I have climbed several mountains in my life, both metaphorically and in reality, but this particular ascent was so very enjoyable to summit with you, despite suffering quite dizzying altitude sickness at times. For now, let's just enjoy the view. Thank you for believing in me, for messaging me that day in May 2022, and allowing me to fulfil a dream and a passion project. In the process, you have helped me heal some deep wounds, and I hope this project gives hope and guidance to so many others who find themselves in a similar predicament as me. A huge thank you to the team at Sheldon Press, John Murray Press and Hachette, including Alisha Raj and Gracie Maddison, for taking me under your wing and supporting my vision for this book.

To my Colorectal Nurse Specialist, Angie. I may have been diagnosed with cancer but thankfully I had the best CNS ever to see me through! Thank you for all your support and encouragement, both during and beyond my cancer treatment, you have been my lifeline, my confidante, and my friend, and I cannot thank you enough.

And of course, to Professor Rockall, the surgeon who saved my life, and who continues to ensure my ongoing health and wellbeing, my words can do little to express the debt of gratitude I owe you. Thank you for both continuing to encourage and support me in all my pursuits, and for agreeing to come on board with this book. Thank you both for your unwavering dedication in the fight against bowel cancer, and for continually striving to better the care of those afflicted by it.

To Danni, once my therapist and now my friend, thank you for being incredible at what you do, and for helping me get back up when I fell so far down. There are not many people that you instantly 'connect' with, but I think the feeling was mutual that fateful day. It's been amazing to reconnect so far along this road, and work together in a professional capacity with me no longer the patient! I know your expertise has helped, and will continue to help, so many.

To my oncologist, Dr Alex Stewart – thank you for guiding me through some tricky decisions, and for the drugs that mopped up any rogue cancer cells which may have been hanging around after surgery. Thank you for being so encouraging with this book, and for providing your esteemed peer review. Your attention to detail is second to none. Through you, I have learnt so much more about the beast, and thank you, too, for your dedication to the cause.

I will always hold the team who gave me life in the highest possible regard. I don't have the words to express my lifelong gratitude, but to each and every one of you, including the countless others who have assisted me along the way (too many to name), please know that I am forever indebted to you, and I thank you unreservedly.

Also, a huge thank you to Dr Katie Snape, Consultant Clinical Geneticist, for her invaluable advice and guidance, and for her support and dedication to assisting me in demystifying the world of cancer genetics, I've learnt so much.

I'd also like to thank Barbara Wilson from Working with Cancer for reviewing my piece on returning to work with her expert eyes in this field.

To all the real-life contributors and expert patients, thank you, thank you, thank you from the bottom of my heart for so generously and selflessly sharing your stories, which I know will help others. You fill so many with hope; thank you so much for being part of this moment with me.

Without the contributions from my healthcare professionals, real life contributors and friends, there would be no book. It is you who validate this book, and make it accurate, real, and authentic for others, and I can't begin to express how grateful I am to you all.

To the social media community and Instagram, for always supporting me through the highs and the lows, I never knew such strong connections could be forged with people you've never even met! And I never appreciated the strength one can draw from social media platforms, but I have a loyal following who have encouraged me every step of the way, and I wish to thank them too. I'd also like to take this opportunity to also acknowledge and thank all the cancer community past and present who've supported me, who've taught me and who've stuck by me, as well as the legend that was and still is, the late Dame Deborah James – a beacon of light who showed us how to really live, to find the best in life, to make change and have "no regrets". She has massively influenced a change in the public perception of bowel cancer in the UK and driven awareness. She had a huge influence on me since my diagnosis and gave us all so much hope - I miss her lead, and we all miss her presence dearly, but I've heard her voice in my head on repeated occasions whilst writing this book, chivvying me on to keep going.

A huge thank you to Katie Wooley for getting me started on this adventure and giving me a crash course into the world of publishing and who has kept me going quietly in the background throughout. And to all of you writers for giving me supportive and sound advice, including Liz O'Riordan, Emma Campbell, and Dr Amir Khan. And to Jez Willy for helping me out with a key ingredient of this book too! Thank you.

To the charities I work with – Teens Unite, the Fountain Centre, Bowel Cancer UK, Cancer Research UK – thank you for allowing me a voice, and helping me find my way after cancer, and turn this negative I was dealt with into a positive. It has been an absolute privilege to be part of your campaigns and to be part of the work you carry out, and I'm so grateful for the support you have shown me with my work, including this book.

To my surgery, work colleagues and friends there, thank you for helping make my return to work as painless as possible, supporting me, allowing me to flourish and grow in all directions post cancer and embracing the whirlwind that I indeed am. To the ITV Lorraine team and Helen, for 'seeing something in me' that I just couldn't post cancer, building my confidence and being part of my recovery, allowing me a platform and outlet to talk all things cancer, health and taboo busting. You've helped me fulfil what I hoped and set out to achieve as soon as I was diagnosed. I'm forever grateful.

I'd also like to thank my brothers, Kayur and Rishi for always allowing me to boss them around as their older and wiser sister, (even more so when I had cancer) and for all the help, support and love you have given the four of us with your wonderful wives Lynsey and Abby, especially during cancer. There is no doubt that cancer brought us even closer together, even though we may be miles apart. And I love you all.

To my mum and dad, thank you for encouraging me to push boundaries and for allowing me to bloom into the person I am today. For believing in me, for supporting me (and the children) and showing us how to make the most of life whilst growing up. And thank you to my parents in law, and for their unwavering support through treatment and stepping in on the 'bad' weeks and weekends.

And finally, to my fabulous husband G, thank you for always being there, for guiding me, supporting me and looking after me through the good, the bad and the very ugly. I'm in awe of the fact you continue to do the job that you do, day in, day out, after everything we have been through. You are most definitely my hero, and I am very proud of you. Thank you for your Herculean assistance in helping me write this book, and for encouraging me in all my ventures new. You've got your wife back now, albeit only temporarily...till the next project!

Plenty more adventures to come!

Love you to the moon and back.

Anisha x

Patient Contributors

Andrea Robson	Gemma Collier
Neil Barker	Nat Woodward
Dirren Patel	Stan Jewell
Faith Windsor	Olivia Rowlands
Lauren Fresa	Claire Sharp
Emma Campbell	Sophie Umhofer

Contents

About the author

Dr Anisha Patel MBChB, MRCP, DFSRH, DRCOG, MRCGP undertook her medical training at the University of Birmingham and is now a general practitioner in West Sussex. She is married to a Consultant Gastroenterologist and lives with her family in Surrey, in the UK.

Anisha received the bombshell diagnosis of bowel cancer at the age of 39. Since then, her energy has been focused on raising awareness of bowel cancer, initially through her popular Instagram platform, @doctorsgetcancertoo. Today, she is a speaker and health educator, working as an on-screen doctor across a variety of media outlets to highlight a broad range of health agendas. Anisha appears regularly on ITV's *Lorraine*, and has appeared on BBC and ITV news and TalkTV, and in podcasts, magazines and print media, breaking health taboos and talking all things health and women's health, with a particular focus on cancers. She has featured on the 'No Butts' campaign, founded by the team from television's *Lorraine*, and the late Dame Deborah James, whose aim is to dispel the stigmas surrounding bowel cancer. Anisha has taken part in a variety of health and cancer-related campaigns, including for the NHS, and for charities, working alongside them and developing a unique perspective as both patient and doctor. She is a Trustee of Teens Unite and a Patron of the Fountain Centre, Guildford, two cancer charities supporting patients from diagnosis, through treatment, and beyond.

Anisha is passionate about, and has significant experience of, talking about survivorship and life after cancer. She devotes much of her spare time to helping others navigate this most difficult, and often not spoken about, phase of life, including how to return to work, and finding a 'new normal'.

Everything You Hoped You'd Never Need to Know About Colorectal Cancer is her debut book.

Foreword

Cancer is common and bowel cancer specifically is one of the most common cancers for men and women. Fortunately, the taboo nature of this diagnosis is gradually becoming a thing of the past and it is a condition much more talked about in the media than ever before. There remain, however, educational and cultural barriers that still need to be overcome. The role of the medical profession, the national bowel cancer screening programme as well as high-profile patients and patient advocates in the media have been hugely important in changing the public understanding and perception of this condition. Although it can be a devastating diagnosis for our patients we have the fortune and privilege of treating a common malignant condition that is often curable – especially if we can diagnose it early.

As a surgeon treating this condition every day it is easy to forget what a potentially huge impact the diagnosis has on the patients and their families. The volume of information in this book tells you much about the tsunami of questions and concerns that accompany the diagnosis and the whole treatment journey that these patients experience.

Anisha and her husband are both doctors and so she has both her own knowledge and experience to draw on and easy access to more specialist knowledge. But despite this she is first and foremost a patient, like any other person with a diagnosis of rectal cancer. Anisha tells her own story from first symptoms to diagnosis and all the way through her treatment and into recovery. The book addresses the technicalities as well as the functional issues, side effects and emotional consequences in a very honest and approachable manner that will be immensely helpful not only to anyone with bowel cancer but also to their family, friends, and carers.

The treatment of colorectal cancer has improved greatly over the last few decades with the introduction of screening, improvements in diagnosis, endoscopy, radiology, surgery, anaesthesia, perioperative care, stoma care and oncology as well as a better understanding of the genetics of the disease. At the same time, the care of patients now involves a complex process of decision making, involving a multi-disciplinary team that oversees the management of each individual patient. Most patients, however, will still come to surgery – and this, too, has changed beyond recognition. Historically surgery for bowel cancer was a significant trauma to the patients – involving major abdominal surgery, a prolonged stay in hospital, and a long recovery. Today, many patients can benefit from minimally invasive (keyhole) techniques and improved perioperative care leading to a shorter stay in hospital, fewer complications and a more rapid return to normal activity. In the future, advances in our understanding of the genetics and the biology of the disease will help us better identify the patients at higher risk and, with appropriate screening, develop preventative strategies and enable us to detect even more cases at a pre-malignant or early stage of the disease.

Anisha's contribution to increasing public awareness of bowel cancer and to helping patients deal with this common disease is both significant and admirable. She has written a hugely useful book that makes a great contribution to the literature available to our patients.

Professor Tim Rockall
Consultant Surgeon, Royal Surrey NHS Foundation Trust Guildford
Professor of Surgery, University of Surrey
Director of the Minimal Access Training Unit (MATTU), Guildford

Prologue

We all have dates that carry particular significance.

Our children's birthdays, our anniversaries, our noteworthy achievements, perhaps.

For G and I, 21 September 2018 is one of ours.

The date that cancer was diagnosed.

When the earth stopped spinning.

And time stood still.

Because I'll let you in on a secret.

Einstein got it wrong.

Time has nothing to do with matter. Or the speed of light. Contrary to popular opinion, the space–time continuum can, in fact, be warped quite easily.

You see, to make time come to a grinding, juddering, gut-wrenching halt, you just need to hear the words, 'You have cancer'... And all of time that precedes that moment – all your memories of a happier, healthier, cancer-free life – is ripped from beneath your feet with such force it leaves you spinning.

It's as if a massive cancer black hole suddenly opens up right next to you, inexorably sucking your pre-cancer life deep into its black abyss.

You're instantly catapulted into another dimension – an alternative existence. Cancer omnipresent. And life in this parallel cancer universe doesn't obey the laws of physics either – here, time continues to seemingly bend and flex, slowing right down in the run-up to test results, and going 'blink-and-you'll-miss-it' quick during breaks between chemo.

And if space rocks were side-effects, then the asteroid-belt of chemotherapy is vast. Negotiating it, perilously dangerous. Head-on collisions, unavoidable. And when they happen, you don't break, you bounce, from one rock to another, your protective shield progressively cracked and weakened with each subsequent impact.

And if we make it through, the weeks of travelling will no doubt take their toll.

Some damage sustained.

Inevitable.

Irreparable.

And we may then find ourselves confronted by a new blackness, disorientated and directionless, consumed by a gnawing, unassuaged and primal fear, of the unknown, of what lies ahead in uncharted territory … But we will make it through.

I know this with certainty.

Because just as Einstein had a constant, so we do too.

Our children.

Our beautiful, amazing children.

We are so blessed.

Over these past few years our children have been the most phenomenal little human beings you could ever have the pleasure of knowing. They have demonstrated such resilience and tenacity, and displayed such love and affection, through these, the most challenging times we have faced in their short lives, it has been nothing short of astonishing.

They have been with us since the beginning.

They travel with us wherever we go.

And THEY are our unbreakable shield.

So, $E = mc^2$, where 'c' stands for children.

Sorry, Albert.

GJS, December 2018

Introduction

Colorectal cancer (CRC), or bowel cancer as it is also known, is the third most common cancer diagnosed in both sexes in the Western world. It is also the second biggest cancer killer. Every 15 minutes, somebody is diagnosed with bowel cancer in the UK. My 15-minute appointment was scheduled for 21 September 2018.

Young, old, female or male, every colour and every culture, it takes no prisoners.

And the impact upon all those around the individual diagnosed is colossal. I never in a million years understood quite the level of devastation and heartache it could cause, not only at diagnosis and through treatment, but also during life after cancer. We can become so focused on the negatives, but I also hadn't fully appreciated the positives that it could gift you either.

Everyone's cancer experience is unique, however, and this is extremely important to remember throughout this book.

Why write a book?

I've been to medical school, I've studied hard my entire life, yet no amount of grafting could have prepared me for the shit storm that is cancer. My learning curve was exponential, not only from my personal experiences, but also from what I learnt through my own research, from what I've observed from the experience of others within the cancer community, and from the insight and opinions of health professionals I've met along the way. My brain has been a sponge, squirrelling away every nugget of information – be it factual or something related to emotional intelligence, it has changed my clinical practice forever. There are some gems that I've collected along the way, gems I wish I'd known beforehand that would have explained a whole host of emotions and issues and would have reassured me that a lot of what I experienced was in fact completely normal. These gems need to be shared among the wider population, and this is my aim, and why a lot of this book is applicable to all cancers, not just bowel cancer.

I fully appreciate that just because I'm a doctor and I've had bowel cancer, it doesn't make me an expert on 'everything you hoped you'd never need to know about colorectal cancer'. So, I've brought on board a whole host of professionals, many of whom have been involved in my care; my consultant colorectal surgeon, Professor Timothy Rockall, my consultant oncologist, Dr Alexandra Stewart, my husband, who happens to be a consultant gastroenterologist, Dr Gareth Sadler, my cancer specialist nurse, Angie Bates, a consultant clinical geneticist, Dr Katie Snape, and my counsellor and psychotherapist, Danielle Freeth. In addition to their wealth of expertise, I have drafted in some other big guns, and these are the people with the knowledge of a *lived* experience of bowel cancer who have offered to come on board from the bowel cancer community, and I'm honoured and grateful for them to have shared some of their stories and insight with you, so candidly.

As you read through this book, my expert team and I would like to help you steer your way through the pandemonium that is cancer and, for those diagnosed with or who have a loved one diagnosed with bowel cancer, may it become your companion and your hope. You may choose to read it in its entirety or dip in and out as you please, if indeed you have the misfortune of entering the chaotic and overwhelming world of cancer. Even though you will hopefully have an army of support behind you, cancer can be an extremely lonely place, and having an ear that 'just gets it' is so, so vital. For those that are reading this and have not been touched by cancer, I hope you find it educational, entertaining at times and insightful.

'Life after cancer' is a whole different entity in many ways and the latter half of the book is dedicated to this. It's a huge period of adjustment and can be equally as tough, if not tougher, than treatment itself, and there is definitely a reason people sometimes quote 'Cancer, the gift that keeps on giving'. During this part of my cancer experience, it was apparent that there was a colossal void needing to be filled with support and conversations regarding the aftermath of cancer, a subject I feel passionate talking about openly and honestly. I'm hoping to share the highs and the lows, as well as highlight any learning points and helpful tips to aid the process of recovery, healing and growth during this phase.

When I was diagnosed, there wasn't a book that could cover everything from the time of diagnosis to life after cancer, with all the medical and psychological bits in between, that I *really* wanted to know. I was handed literature from various forums but felt totally bewildered by the endless array of pamphlets that greeted me at every hospital visit and which I would neatly file away. Even being a doctor, the information just wasn't processing.

This book offers a wealth of knowledge about not only bowel cancer, but also life after (any) cancer, with my team and I holding your hand all the way.

For now, I'll start by introducing myself and my story, and throughout the book you will discover vignettes of my experience, as well as the experience of others, to bring to life the world of bowel cancer and beyond.

About me, my diagnosis, and why I am so passionate about this book

Hi, I'm Anisha.

I was diagnosed with stage 3B rectal cancer, aged 39.

I am a general practitioner (GP) with specialist interests in women's health, respiratory medicine and now cancer awareness, health education and health promotion. Some may call me a campaigner for cancer awareness. I honestly just want to make whatever difference in whatever capacity I can, big or small, to push the agenda for cancer awareness and health and to help those that find themselves on this uphill treadmill. This all started off on a social media platform, which my best friend encouraged me to set up (@doctorsgetcancertoo), which early on became a platform for my own catharsis and journalling, but also for community and supporting others, and later developed into a platform to document my recovery, raise awareness and offer health education for all.

I volunteer for charities such as Bowel Cancer UK and Cancer Research UK in a media volunteer capacity as both a doctor and a patient, as an ethnic minority voicing the health inequalities we may face and looking always for ways we may be able to help. More recently, I was appointed as a Trustee of Teens Unite in 2022, a teenage cancer charity – whose aim is to help support young patients through diagnosis and treatment as well as help them navigate their way through life after cancer and beyond, with their return to work and education. I advise on their board as both a doctor and patient, something that is hugely fulfilling and which is a passion project in itself. I was also honoured to take up the role as a patron for the wonderful charity that is the Fountain Centre this year, a holistic cancer centre, that my family and I accessed, which I'll talk about in more detail later.

Somewhere along the line, whilst navigating life after cancer, I ended up working in the media and as a TV doctor (and patient advocate), raising awareness not only of cancer but also for a variety of topics and news items. It is an opportunity that I relish and thrive upon, knowing there is a huge platform to impart information from and that it is an opportunity I may never have had, were it not for cancer.

My family. I have two beautiful, heartwarming children, full of boundless energy, who at the time of diagnosis were aged six and seven. It broke my heart when I was diagnosed, knowing the cancer ripples would soon reach their shores, and cascade to all those around, knowing that our lives would never be the same again. The uncertainty that they have had to live with from such a young age weighs heavy on my shoulders but, as children often do, they see me as invincible. My husband, G, is a consultant gastroenterologist and was at the time of diagnosis one of the regional leads for the UK's National Bowel Cancer Screening Programme. He is now the lead for the endoscopy service at his London-based teaching hospital. He spends most of his time trying to diagnose bowel cancer at an early stage, as well as treating early bowel cancers and polyps (some of which will be precancerous) using highly specialized procedures. He is also, very much, my unshakeable rock.

I remember the earliest discussions with my husband included how I wished my diagnosis to be shared. Of course, everyone is individual, but I felt compelled to be open and honest about my diagnosis, which is hopefully reflected in this book. As doctors, we have a huge desire to use my experience and platform to help others and their loved ones through their own cancer experiences, should they find themselves in this gut-wrenching position. I've been there, and I have many T-shirts to match the host of trials and tribulations that cancer brings, and I'm hoping to share some of my wardrobe with you.

I have also talked a lot about creating positivity out of the negative hand that we were dealt. One thing high on our agenda was to ensure we help raise awareness, among both health professionals and the public, of bowel cancer in the young, as we know that those diagnosed young are often diagnosed at a later stage of cancer. We are keen to help alleviate the frequently encountered stigmas surrounding this cancer, and bowel cancer screening, by sharing our story. This is in a bid to try to stop people presenting late to health professionals by encouraging them to get checked early, and attending screening appointments. Because what we do know is that EARLY DIAGNOSIS SAVES LIVES.

We know there are so many inspiring people out there going through this, confronting their own tough journey day by day, step by step, and who may be championing this cause, many of whom have helped and supported me through my time with cancer and continue to do so. Together with my health professionals, friends, family, and the online community who support my visions, embrace my enthusiasm, my crazy, my passions, my hopes and dreams, and who have helped me live my life to the fullest I possibly can post cancer, I just wanted to start by saying 'Thank you'.

I am forever grateful.

Anisha.

My story

'It's nasty.'

These were the very words which were imparted to me at diagnosis as my groggy mind, pumped full of sedative and morphine, tried to make sense of what I could see on the screen. A bloody mass presented in high definition, in all its glory, being tugged apart by the biopsy forceps. In retrospect, the room had fallen silent, and phone calls were being made. To the cancer specialist nurse. To the CT scanner for an urgent CT. To my husband. This is the point at which your world disintegrates around you, crashing down with the loudest bang you will ever hear.

The disbelief, of being blind-sided by this meteorite. It seems so foreign.

Yet one in two of us will get cancer.

Being a family doctor, one could say I should have known better. But I felt sure that my symptoms could have been attributable to piles and irritable bowel syndrome (IBS). I was, and would like to think I still am, a fit and healthy individual with no risk factors and no family history of any cancer. I didn't look or feel unwell, having completed an 8 km assault course only the weekend before. But with the benefit of hindsight, things maybe were just not quite right ...

If I go back to the beginning and set the scene, I probably had what I thought were new-onset IBS symptoms approximately nine months before my diagnosis – constipation requiring laxatives intermittently, some urgency in needing to go to the toilet, and occasionally some fresh blood on the toilet paper. But since childbirth six years ago, a little blood every now and again on the toilet paper from a previous pile was not that unusual.

Tiredness was also a feature, but I expected nothing less as a part-time doctor, mother of two energetic children, running a household and, quite frankly, I can't remember the last time I wasn't tired. I had seen my GP for that reason nine months prior to diagnosis and all my blood tests were normal then, and things were left at that point, with nobody thinking any more of it.

Four months prior to diagnosis, the constipation and occasional blood on the toilet paper were becoming more intrusive. I started to experience an increasing feeling of incomplete bowel emptying (like I hadn't finished a poo properly) after I'd gone to the toilet. The blood became more noticeable, initially on the paper, but then in the pan, and in July 2018 my bowel habit was, for want of a better expression, frankly explosive. I knew that something was wrong. I finally spoke to my husband about my symptoms as I felt that things weren't settling. We both agreed I would go to the doctor to seek further help.

By this point, the summer holidays were in full swing, I had been examined and further blood tests had been requested. I commenced a prescription for regular laxatives and suppositories for presumed piles and possible IBS, and actually I thought my symptoms slightly improved. However, by the end of August whilst we were having our family holiday in Italy, things became progressively worse. I noticed that I was really quite fatigued. I was tiring and short of breath when running shorter distances than usual, I honestly felt like a sloth running backwards. I decided it was the effects of the scorching conditions I was attempting to run in, so thought nothing more. I was treating myself to afternoon siestas, and then falling asleep by eight thirty each night, apparently messaging friends about how fatigued I felt. Despite indulging in every Italian carbohydrate possible, looking back at pictures now, I am convinced I started looking slimmer, despite eating more lavishly while abroad. I found myself rushing to the toilet in the early hours of the morning and on the final day, the blood spatter in the pan was alarming. I braved showing my husband and from the look on his face, I knew immediately I had to go back to my doctor. Our medical theory at this point was that I may have some sort of inflammatory bowel disease. My husband and I were obviously fully aware of colorectal cancer in the under-50s – we'd had many conversations about the number of (anonymous) cases that were presenting in this age group over recent years (you're never too young) – never thinking I would be one of them.

When I saw the doctor on my return, I explained the progression of my symptoms and requested a referral. My recent bloods had come back as showing I was also anaemic, something I'd suffered with on and off through my life due to my periods, but I no longer had periods due to a coil being fitted. This anaemia was most likely to be coming from the blood loss I was experiencing from my gut. The doctor and I agreed for a referral to be made through our urgent suspected cancer pathway that exists in the UK – called a 'two-week wait' referral. This ensures that patients have their first initial consultation with a specialist within two weeks of the referral being sent off.

Even when I saw the colorectal surgeon, the working diagnosis was 'functional IBS and piles' on his letter. In the ten days I waited for my colonoscopy, the bleeding was becoming worrisome and it had increased in volume and frequency. One night, I had an episode of such severe abdominal pain I nearly called an ambulance.

The day of my colonoscopy, I was fully expecting a diagnosis of piles, colitis, something – but not cancer. That poor surgeon was confronted by my tumour the minute the colonoscope entered my rectum, and from that moment, all conversation halted in the room.

In rapid succession, soon after I was told it was 'nasty', I underwent a variety of further investigations. First, I underwent a staging CT scan to look for evidence of cancer spread (known as metastases), to my liver and lungs, which I thankfully didn't have. I had also been experiencing sciatica for several weeks prior, with no previous history of any similar symptoms. Sciatica can be a feature of rectal cancer, so obviously we were concerned that the tumour may have spread locally into my spine.

Waiting for my pelvic and spinal MRI scan to assess the situation further was the longest four days of my life, but thankfully there was no evidence of spread – but I did have a prolapsed disc to add to the list of diagnoses!

When all the necessary tests were complete, I was told I had a diagnosis of stage 3C (locally advanced) rectal cancer.

Even 30 minutes after the bombshell was dropped, some of my first conversations with my husband were that I wanted two important things. First, to be open about my diagnosis, my symptoms and my treatment plan with our friends and families. I had nothing to hide. It was nothing to be ashamed of. I wanted people to be aware that it could happen to anyone and never take anything for granted. And importantly, I wanted to know that my family and I had the support I knew we would need to guide us through the eye of the storm, and beyond.

Secondly, I also wanted to maintain as much normality in my life, especially for my children. So with this in mind, I continued to make plans for a planned trip to Sierra Nevada with seven extremely supportive friends, to climb the highest mountain in Spain – Mount Mulhacen – the following week. I was determined not to let cancer start controlling my life already, nor did I want it to get in my way. My surgeon was brilliantly supportive of this decision and arranged for surgery to be scheduled on my return.

I finally received clearance to continue with the trip 12 hours before we were due to fly and it was the best decision I ever made. Although I didn't summit to 3500 m on medical advice due to the altitude and my anaemia causing me severe breathlessness, I completed most of the three-day trek and reached 3250 metres above sea level. I knew on my return I had a much bigger mountain to climb so was absolutely one hundred per cent determined to get this one under my belt beforehand!

However, in the quest to carry on with life as usual in the lead up to my operation, I began to suffer panic attacks at night. I was seemingly fine, keeping busy and distracted in the day. However, at night the demon subconscious would appear, and I didn't sleep properly in the weeks leading up to the op. The cumulative exhaustion proved very limiting, and before long I had to stop working as a doctor, a job that I really loved. As I had not experienced a panic attack before, I initially thought I might be having a pulmonary embolism (a blood clot in the lung that people with cancer are more likely to develop). And as a long list of other possible medical explanations for my symptoms started playing repeatedly in my head, I realized that my medical training might be a double-edged sword on my long journey ahead.

After seeing the doctor again, I spoke to the colorectal nurse, Angie, who was just fantastic, and, although I didn't know it at first, she would become a lifeline from day one. She signposted me to an amazing holistic centre attached to the cancer unit, the Fountain Centre. Little did I know how invaluable they would become in the months ahead, for both me and my family. I had some hypnotherapy sessions, too, which helped alleviate my anxiety symptoms.

In October 2018, I underwent an operation, initially an examination under anaesthetic, to assess whether my cancer was operable. I found contemplating the prospect of surgery tremendously nerve-wracking, and the uncertainty about whether my surgeon would be able to excise the cancer or not played havoc with my mind in the long days leading up to my surgical D-day, only serving to heighten my anxiety further.

On account of the size of my tumour, it also wasn't clear-cut whether the chances of it being removed surgically would be increased by a course of neoadjuvant chemo-radiotherapy (treatment given *before* surgery to increase the chances of surgery being successful). The surgeon and oncologist involved both my husband and me in the decision-making processes, and we decided to pursue the surgical approach first, as this might possibly spare me the chemo-radiotherapy and all the potential side effects that come hand in hand with this treatment, assuming the tumour could be removed successfully at operation.

I've never felt fear like it, adrenaline pumping through my veins, the day I was wheeled into the operating room with the anaesthetist. I was feeling out of control – my place wasn't on the patient trolley, it should be as the doctor! So vulnerable. It felt so wrong. I was sedated through tears as I went under general anaesthetic, not knowing what I was going to wake up to – the cancer gone and perhaps a stoma, or the cancer still there and needing chemo-radiotherapy before they could even entertain the tumour being removed.

However, my tumour was (thankfully) deemed operable, and I underwent a laparoscopic anterior resection and a total mesenteric excision. The decision was made to give me a temporary ileostomy (stoma) from a surgical safety perspective, to allow the surgical join to heal where the tumour had been removed.

My husband tells me that time stood still for him as he paced the corridors in the hours I was away from him in theatre. I, on the other hand, woke up bleary-eyed in the recovery room with beeping machines surrounding me, unaware of my fate. My hand slowly moved towards my belly, knowing I had to firstly find out whether surgery had taken place and secondly, whether there was a stoma. Through the curtain my surgeon's head appeared. He smiled, the tumour was gone, removed in its entirety, and the relief was palpable.

Yet this was just the beginning.

PART 1
DIAGNOSIS AND TREATMENT OF COLORECTAL CANCER

1

Colorectal cancer – what do I need to know?

Come and meet the large bowel

The large bowel

The large bowel is made up of the colon, the rectum and the anal canal. Food passes from the stomach into the small intestine (where essentially nutrients are absorbed) and then on to the colon.

The colon

The function of the colon is then to absorb most of the water and salt from the remaining digested food, which progressively solidifies as it passes through the colon, eventually being stored in the rectum as poo/stool.

The rectum

The rectum is the storage vessel for stools (poop, or poo) and links the colon to the anus as you can see from Figure 1.1. It is about 15 cm long. The rectum is divided into three parts: the upper, middle and lower thirds. The rectum stretches as it fills with poo, and this stretch lets the brain know when we need to defecate or open our bowels. Nerves and muscles can help us hold on to stools until we find a convenient time and place to pass it through the opening at the end of the large bowel, called the anal canal.

The anal canal

The anal canal is approximately 4 cm long and has a nerve supply which allows us to distinguish whether the urge to pass is related to wind or poo (an absolutely vital and ingenious design!). The anal sphincter is a ring of muscles which opens and closes to allow bowel movements to pass under conscious control. Disorders of the anal canal or damage to its nerve supply can result in incontinence.

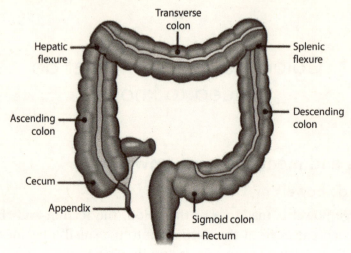

Figure 1.1 Anatomy of the large bowel
Source: Bowel Cancer UK

What is a normal stool and a normal bowel habit?

Firstly, everyone is different! When it comes to bowel habit, there simply is no 'normal'. A healthy bowel movement (stool) should be pain free to pass and require minimal straining. Some people may defecate three times a day, others three times a week. This spectrum is normal if you have always been this way inclined.

What is essential to appreciate, however, is what constitutes a normal bowel habit for YOU, and even more importantly, that when you notice a persistent change (usually defined as a period of more than three weeks) away from your normal, you seek early medical advice.

Figure 1.2 shows the Bristol Stool Chart developed as a clinical assessment tool in 1997 by Ken Heaton, which patients find a particularly helpful communication aid in describing their stools. It is used by doctors to diagnose certain conditions such as constipation, and monitors the effectiveness of treatments for bowel diseases. Crucially, it also allows doctors and patients to identify more objectively if there has been a persistent change in bowel habit that may require further investigation. Commonly, one in 12 of a general practitioner's consultations will be regarding a gastrointestinal issue, so in day-to-day practice, this is a really useful tool.

The Bristol Stool Chart classifies the different states of stool. Types 3 and 4 are considered 'healthy'. Types 1 and 2 represent constipation, while types 5, 6 and 7 are more towards the diarrhoea end of the spectrum.

Bristol Stool Chart

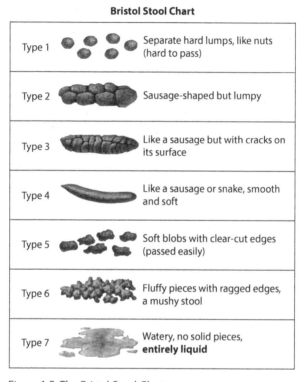

Type 1	Separate hard lumps, like nuts (hard to pass)
Type 2	Sausage-shaped but lumpy
Type 3	Like a sausage but with cracks on its surface
Type 4	Like a sausage or snake, smooth and soft
Type 5	Soft blobs with clear-cut edges (passed easily)
Type 6	Fluffy pieces with ragged edges, a mushy stool
Type 7	Watery, no solid pieces, **entirely liquid**

Figure 1.2 The Bristol Stool Chart

The colour of your stool is determined partly by your diet, and partly by how much bile it contains. Bile is produced in the gall bladder and is a yellow-green fluid that contains enzymes to digest fats. A poo which is any shade of brown or even green is considered normal.

Blood in the stool is NOT normal.

I am absolutely convinced that, by talking more openly about our bowel habits, teaching our children about bodily functions and calling body parts by their correct anatomical names, patients will feel less embarrassment or shame to seek help from their doctor in the event they encounter a persistent change from their normal.

Checking your poo before you flush, and checking the toilet tissue after wiping, should be encouraged. This may help identify bleeding, and changes in your stool form or consistency. If these occur, it does not mean you have bowel cancer, but you should not delay a consult with your doctor for further advice and assessment.

What is colorectal cancer (CRC)?

Colorectal cancer is also known as bowel cancer. It is a term that covers cancer of the colon (colon cancer) or cancer of the rectum (rectal cancer). Most colorectal cancers arise from a benign growth of the inner lining of the colon or rectum known as a *polyp*.

Most colorectal cancers are adenocarcinomas – these start in the cells that produce mucus to lubricate the inside of the colon and rectum – but there are other types of cancers occurring in the bowel which are much rarer, including lymphomas, sarcomas, melanomas, carcinoids and gastrointestinal stromal tumours (GISTs).

The development of a bowel cancer from a polyp (see Figure 6.1) is a slow process (usually occurring over many years) and it is thought that, overall, only about 5 per cent of polyps become malignant (cancerous) over time, so who knows how long my cancer had been growing! The vast majority of polyps that are benign therefore remain benign, but there is currently no way of predicting which will do so. It really is a polyp lottery. Polyps are usually removed if found at colonoscopy, and this helps significantly reduce the risk of developing colorectal cancer, but does not completely protect against it. If you have previously had polyps removed but develop a persistent change in your bowel habit, or bleeding, you should still seek medical advice.

What are the symptoms of colorectal cancer?

The acronym BOWEL is an easy way to remember and share the symptoms of bowel cancer.

- **B**lood in your stool or from your bottom
- **O**bvious change in bowel habit (persistent for more than three weeks)
- **W**eight loss for no apparent reason

- Extreme tiredness
- Lump in the tummy or pain in the tummy

If you or a loved one have any of these signs or symptoms, AND they are persistent, please do not delay in seeing your GP or family doctor.

There are other symptoms (in addition to those above) which can be a sign of rectal cancer:

- A sensation of pressure or fullness in the rectum/back passage
- A feeling of incomplete bowel emptying
- Thin or ribbon-like poo
- Urgency to open your bowels, especially at night

I was experiencing all these symptoms by the time I was diagnosed with rectal cancer. I also experienced two bouts of severe abdominal pain which lasted for several hours ('call the ambulance' type of pain), but which settled spontaneously, so I thought nothing more of it.

I'm so embarrassed – how do I tell my doctor I have a problem 'down there'?

Patients often tell me they have been too embarrassed to seek help, or that they are afraid to come and see me with their symptoms because of what I might suggest needs to be done. But please rest assured that the consultation with your doctor is in absolute confidence, and that this work is a doctor's bread and butter – there are probably few things your doctor will have not seen or heard!

With this in mind, I'm going to leave some advice below because I think it's so important to share tips with people who may feel too embarrassed to go to the doctor with a health problem.

Tips: Don't be embarrassed to talk to your doctor

- Firstly, there is never any need to apologize. We want to see you, and help you with whatever problem you're facing.
- Remember your doctor or health professional has probably either seen or heard it all before. This is the nature of our job. We are trained to listen to your history and focus examinations on whichever body part(s) need to be examined, and will formulate a diagnosis or a plan of action. We are NOT distracted by any appearances, odours, body hair or physical appearances.

- Be honest and open about the fact you feel embarrassed so we can do our best to take things at your own pace and address any concerns along the way.
- Book an appointment (if you can) with a member of staff that you bond with, trust or have seen previously.
- Remember your consultation is confidential. There is no judgement.
- Write your symptoms down or keep a symptom diary. You might want to practise what you want to say in front of a mirror.
- Ask questions – so you feel empowered and in control.

In summary, know the symptoms of colorectal cancer, flush away your embarrassment when it comes to talking about poo, know your 'normal', and see your doctor if you have any concerns.

2
Am I at risk?

Risk factors for colorectal cancer

One in 15 men and one in 18 women will be diagnosed with bowel cancer in their lifetime. A person's lifetime risk for developing cancer is complex, and takes into account not just age and genetics but a multitude of other risk factors. What I will start by saying is that if you have a colon or a rectum, you are at risk.

I often get asked, 'So, what caused my bowel cancer?' The answer is, we don't know. For some patients, there are clearly identifiable genetic abnormalities that pre-dispose some to its development, but for most others, it is unlikely to be one single factor, but instead a combination of a multitude of different factors, including diet, ethnicity, genetic make-up, and environment.

I was brought up in a Gujarati household where we seldom ate meat on weekdays, and certainly very little red meat when we did. I thought I was 'fit and healthy'. I exercised several times a week, I wasn't overweight, I am a non-smoker with no family history of bowel cancer, and I was young, and Asian. I was definitely not the stereotypical cancer patient we were taught about at medical school! I just didn't fit the bill, and I didn't think that it could be me. And what this highlights is this – cancer does not discriminate.

We do know, however, that 54 per cent of bowel cancers are potentially preventable through lifestyle changes and lifestyle choices. This is really important to know (whether you have been diagnosed or not) in order to try to prevent this cancer knocking on your door, but also to try to reduce your risk of recurrence if you have already had it. And in any case, the lifestyle measures that are suggested probably reduce the risk of a whole host of other medical conditions as well, so the benefits are likely to extend far beyond cancer prevention!

I firmly believe that everything should be in moderation. So, if you have a penchant for a steak and glass of red wine on a Friday night, go on and treat yourself! Life, after all, is for living. However, I also think it is important to try to achieve a balance. 'But,' I hear you say, '*you* had no risk factors and you were affected by the big C.' Well, that is true, but I still aspire to enjoy my life to its full potential and live well, and I think you can get the balance right with a little thought and planning. If cancer has taught me one thing it is that life is precious, and you only ever have one, so look after it as best you can.

In the section below, I will discuss the risk factors for bowel cancer – those which are modifiable (you can do something about them), and those that are non-modifiable (those which you cannot).

Modifiable lifestyle risk factors for bowel cancer

Red or processed meat

A high consumption can increase your risk of bowel cancer, and 13/100 cases are thought to be linked to a high intake of red or processed meat. Processed meats refers to a meat that has been preserved, smoked, cured or salted. These include: bacon, salami, sausages, hot dogs, ham, tinned meat, beef jerky, or canned meat. Nitrates and nitrites are commonly found in preserved meat and can form carcinogenic compounds (nitrosamines) in the stomach which have been linked to bowel cancer development.

Overcooking, high cooking temperatures, or frying can lead to the generation of advanced glycation end-products (AGES) which are pro-inflammatory and can contribute to the formation of cancer, especially if animal products are involved. This may be linked particularly to early onset colorectal cancer.

The UK government recommends that people eating more than 90 g of red and processed meat a day should reduce it to 70 g or less, and it is important to note that 70 g is the cooked weight. This is equivalent to one and a half sausages, two rashers of thick bacon, five slices of thin lunch ham, half a large burger or five tablespoons of cooked mince.

Suggestions to reduce your intake of red meat or processed meat include:

- Swap red meat for chicken, turkey or fish.
- For mincemeat substitutes, use chicken, turkey or soya mince.
- Use beans, pulses, tofu or paneer.
- Incorporate meat-free days into your weekly meal planner, and perhaps try to view red meat as a 'treat', rather than as a necessity.

Low-fibre diet

Fibre is a plant-based carbohydrate that passes through the body largely undigested, but has a number of health benefits. Research suggests that a low-fibre diet might account for bowel cancer development in approximately 30/100 cases. A huge number!

We are also aware that the average adult ingests only 15–18 g of fibre per day. This means that 9 out of 10 adults in the UK (95 per cent in the US) are not getting enough fibre in their diets.

The daily adult recommendation of fibre is actually 30 g. This intake is actually quite difficult to achieve without actively thinking about it, or specifically meal planning to attain it.

The daily recommendations for fibre intake by age are:

- Age 2–5: 15 g/day
- Age 5–11: 20 g/day
- Age 11–16: 25 g/day
- Adult: 30 g per day

How does a high-fibre diet prevent colorectal cancer?

This is not fully understood, but here are some of the hypotheses:

- Fibre provides a source of 'friendly' bacteria promoting the gut microbiome.
- Fibre aids production of short chain fatty acids which are protective to the gut.
- When fibre meets bacteria in the bowel, it produces a chemical called butyrate. Butyrate helps keep the cells in the bowel healthy, thus preventing cancer.

- Fibre helps us poo more often and reduces the time that stool remains in contact with the bowel lining, reducing its exposure time to any potentially harmful chemicals produced within the gut.

Eating plenty of fibre will not only help reduce your risk of bowel cancer, but has a whole host of other health benefits too, including the following:

- Prevents constipation
- Reduces the risk of stroke
- Reduces the risk of heart disease
- Reduces the risk of developing type 2 diabetes
- Reduces cholesterol
- Improves gut microbiome.

How can I increase the amount of fibre in my diet?

- 'High fibre' foods should have at least 6 g fibre/100 g – so make sure you check the food packaging label.
- Alternatively, a 'source of fibre' food will typically have more than 3 g fibre/100 g.
- Food swaps include:
  o swapping white to brown rice, pasta or bread
  o swapping to whole grain food, cereals, seeds, nuts
  o using pulses, chickpeas, legumes, lentils, or peas as a substitute for meat, either wholly or at least in part.
- Consume fruit and vegetables in good quantity. Try to keep tinned or frozen vegetables or fruit in your cupboard or freezer so there is always this source of fibre available – and don't worry, nutrients are always retained in this form.
- Eat high-fibre snacks (nuts, oatcakes, rye crackers, fruit, vegetable sticks, hummus).
- Ensure you mix fibre from all groups, and think about eating an array of rainbow-coloured foods.
- Add seeds to foods, such as chia seeds, linseeds and flax seeds.
- Increase your fluid intake at the same time as increasing dietary fibre.
- Make sure that when increasing fibre in your diet you start slowly, as increasing fibre rapidly will increase wind, bloating and flatulence, and potentially cause tummy discomfort. This may be significant and

more noticeable if you have undergone previous bowel surgery, have a history of bowel disease or irritable bowel syndrome. Despite slow increases in fibre, I fully appreciate that for some patients, increased dietary fibre, no matter how gently introduced into the diet, can make symptoms worse, and these patients may need to abide by a low-residue, or low-fibre diet (see Appendix) and reintroduce small quantities of fibre slowly over time. This group includes a small sub-set of IBS patients, those with inflammatory bowel disease, and some who have had previous bowel surgery.

Understanding the difference between fibre types can also help us to make informed choices as to which fibre-containing foods to increase and which to decrease depending on the symptoms that may be experienced. There are two main types of fibre – soluble and insoluble. Soluble fibre dissolves in water, but insoluble does not. Most plants contain both types of fibre but in differing proportions.

Soluble fibre is found in a variety of foods including oats, peas, beans, apples, citrus fruits, carrots, barley and psyllium. As it passes through your digestive tract, soluble fibre dissolves and forms a gel-like substance which helps to soften stool and promotes the movement of waste material through your digestive system, so it can be of benefit to those who struggle with constipation, particularly when stools are especially firm, bulky or infrequent.

Insoluble fibre is found in foods such as wheat bran, wholegrains, skins, pips and seeds of fruit and vegetables, raw or uncooked vegetables or fibrous vegetables such as rhubarb and celery. Its main action is to bulk the stool which helps to improve stool form and frequency, particularly in those whose diet is lacking in this type of fibre. These foods often pass through the bowel without being digested or absorbed.

In addition to the above effects, both types of fibre may help to lower cholesterol, and may reduce the risk of developing diabetes.

The bottom line – **increase your dietary fibre if you can!**

Physical inactivity

There is strong evidence to suggest that those who are more physically active have a lower incidence of not only bowel cancer but other cancers too, as well as many other health conditions. Approximately 5 per cent of colorectal cancers are thought to be due to physical inactivity.

The recommendation for physical activity is 150 minutes of moderate activity per week, spread throughout the week. This could include, for example, dancing, gardening, hiking or cycling. Even 75 minutes of vigorous activity a week is thought to reduce your risk – so what are you waiting for? Get running, swimming, gardening, dancing, skipping, playing football, walking or cycling up hills, spinning, circuits, weight lifting ... or whatever takes your fancy, just get moving! It also does wonders for the rest of your physical and mental health!

Obesity

Obesity is thought to account for approximately 11 in every 100 cases of bowel cancer. The risk increases proportionately to the length of time an individual remains overweight and how excessively over-weight they are.

In bowel cancer development, it is thought that excess fat causes an increase in levels of the hormone insulin and other growth factors which signal cells to divide more rapidly, including cancer cells.

Obesity poses a greater risk of colon cancer for men of all ages and for pre-menopausal women than it does for post-menopausal women.

Smoking

The risk of bowel cancer increases in proportion to the number of cigarettes smoked, and is thought to be a potential causative factor in 7 of every 100 cases of bowel cancer.

Alcohol

Alcohol is thought to contribute to approximately 6 out of 100 cases of colorectal cancer.

Moderate to heavy alcohol consumption is associated with a 1.2- to 1.5-fold increased risk of cancers of the colon and rectum compared to individuals with no alcohol consumption.

It is important to highlight here that not everyone who has a low-fibre, high-red-meat diet, who drinks alcohol and smokes, will develop colorectal cancer, but the risk of cancer developing from adopting these lifestyle choices is increased, and can be reduced through even minor lifestyle changes.

Non-modifiable risk factors for bowel cancer

Age

The risk of colorectal cancer increases with age. Nearly 6 out of every 10 cases will be diagnosed in patients over 70, and nearly 9 out of 10 cases in patients over 50.

We also know that you are 'never too young' to develop bowel cancer. I *should* know. Young adults and even teenagers have been diagnosed with this cancer, too. The average age at the time of diagnosis of colon cancer for men is 72 years, and 68 years for women.

There is currently an observable increase in the number of rectal cancers being diagnosed in young women. In the UK, according to Bowel Cancer UK, 2,600 people are diagnosed with cancer each year. To put this into perspective, it is roughly equivalent to the total number of people diagnosed each year with testicular cancer or cervical cancer in the UK.

Ethnicity

White ethnic groups have a higher incidence rate of colorectal cancer than Asian, Black or mixed ethnicity groups.

Inflammatory bowel disease (IBD)

The term IBD broadly includes those patients with a diagnosis of Crohn's or ulcerative colitis (UC), in other words, chronic inflammation of the gastrointestinal tract. Patients with IBD have an increased risk of developing colorectal cancer compared to the general population.

The risk of developing colorectal cancer for people with ulcerative colitis is estimated as 2 per cent after 10 years, 8 per cent after 20 years, and 18 per cent after 30 years of disease. The risk of developing colorectal cancer for people with Crohn's disease is considered to be similar to that for people with ulcerative colitis with the same extent of colon affected by the disease.

Patients with IBD are offered surveillance (which typically involves a colonoscopy every 1–5 years, depending on the individual's risk) so that if bowel cancer does develop it can hopefully be caught at an early stage, which improves outcome.

Below, I'd like you to meet my friend, Andrea, who shares her history of IBD and the subsequent development of bowel cancer at a young age.

Meet Andrea Robson (@goodasgold_akr): ulcerative colitis and bowel cancer
Being diagnosed as a young child in a small northern town back in the 1980s
was tough. It took a long time with multiple GP visits until one doctor finally took
my symptoms seriously and I was referred to a local hospital. After various tests
I was finally diagnosed with (pan) ulcerative colitis aged six.

A form of inflammatory bowel disease, ulcerative colitis is a lifelong diagnosis and has no cure. It affects the lining of the large colon and rectum: your
body basically attacks itself, causing pain, bleeding, urgency, fatigue and
weight loss along with inflammation, ulceration and extra symptoms in the
joints, eyes and skin. The longer you have ulcerative colitis, the higher your
risk of developing bowel cancer. It is still uncommon, but indeed it did happen
to me.

Growing up with UC, I was often in a lot of pain and would go to the toilet
more than 20 times a day or I'd stay on the toilet for hours at a time. Over the
years I took many different medications, was in and out of hospital with weekly
blood tests and far too many colonoscopies (under general anaesthetic due to
my age). However, it didn't stop me. I was small but tough. Despite the many
setbacks I carried on with school, went to dance classes a few times a week – I
was obsessed! I wasn't going to let my illness stop me from doing what I loved
no matter how hard it was.

I was referred to an adult clinic aged 16, a big change in support between
paeds and adult care. I went to university, a couple of hours away from home,
but luckily due to my UC I was given a room with an ensuite in the student halls
for the first year. I did a physical course (dance) and went to classes and lectures,
even in pain and during flare-ups; I was determined to get my degree. After
university I moved to London to become a dancer, then later, an assistant in
the media industry. I had plenty of flare-ups but also had periods of remission,
had regular surveillance, colonoscopies, a few hospital admissions and many
changes in medications.

I had my yearly colonoscopy in January 2016. It showed moderate UC,
not surprising. But in the April I started with a bad flare-up and my symptoms
became increasingly worse over the next few months. My bowel habits were all
over the place, I had increasing pain, bleeding, the fatigue was off the charts (I'd
hide in the work toilets for mini naps). But I plodded on. In the November, I was
on a break in Brighton with my partner, when I realized something wasn't right.
I spoke to my IBD nurse who prescribed a course of steroids, thinking it was a
severe flare-up. I had a gastroenterologist appointment already scheduled for
the following month, so we'd wait to see if the steroids would help. That following weekend I was in so much pain, I couldn't cope anymore, so went to A&E.
I was admitted and ten days later (still an inpatient) I heard those dreaded words:
'Andrea, you have cancer.' Wow. My consultant and his team were shocked just
as much as I was.

My surgery was in January 2017, a sub total colectomy with end ileostomy
(the whole colon was removed to reduce the risk of future colon cancer). RIP to
my large colon and hello to my designer bag. Eight months of chemotherapy

followed. Since then, I've had many a scare and plenty of hospital admissions, four emergency surgeries with a bit of sepsis thrown in, now wear two stoma bags (due to a hole forming in my pelvis aka a fistula) and another major surgery is incoming.

I had no visible signs of cancer in January 2016, the biopsies showed no dysplasia (cancer cells forming). But within ten months I had a large tumour at my splenic flexure. By surgery time it had grown more, broken through my bowel wall and attached itself to my spleen, giving me a T4B mucinous adeno-carcinoma tumour. I named it Jabba the Hut. So, my advice for any IBD patients (UC or Crohn's) is:

- Keep a check on your symptoms.
- Know your IBD 'normal'.
- Keep a symptoms journal.
- Keep your clinic appointments.
- Keep going for your regular colonoscopies.
- Keep taking your medication.
- If something doesn't feel right, call your IBD nurse, email your gastro until you're investigated.
- Most importantly, keep being you.

People say 'don't let your illness define your life'. For me, who's had a chronic illness from such a young age and then cancer – well, it kind of has. It's made me the person I am today and I'm proud of me. I'm grateful for the care I've received and when those down times hit, I remind myself that.

UC, in a roundabout way, has helped me get through my bowel cancer life. I was already in the hospital system, luckily. My resilience was high, in that I was used to doctors, cannulas and cameras up my bum. This helped me get through the physical aspects and treatment of bowel cancer. Mentally it was tougher, but it also made me realize how poorly I'd been throughout my life.

Always remember: You've Got This.

The genetics of bowel cancer

Heritable factors account for approximately 35 per cent of colorectal cancer risk, and almost 30 per cent of the population in the UK have a family history of CRC. Five to ten per cent of all CRC cases are thought to be due to genetic mutations (a change in the gene, increasing the risk of bowel cancer, which can then be passed down to other family members). There are also genetic syndromes which increase the risk of colorectal cancer.

I'd like you to meet my family friend, Dirren, diagnosed with stage 2 bowel cancer age 28, long before I was, and the first person I went to visit after my diagnosis. He shares his story of being diagnosed with Lynch syndrome, the most common cause of hereditary CRC.

Dirren (@pateldirren)

I had an open right-sided colectomy in August 2013. No further chemotherapy was needed as there was thankfully no spread to any lymph nodes. The analysis of the tumour did however suggest a genetic condition called Lynch syndrome (see below) was possible and a further blood test confirmed the changes in the tumour were in fact due to an inherited MLH1 change. Suddenly, it all made sense. Cancer has been rife on my father's side of the family. No testing had been offered to anyone in the family prior to my diagnosis. Being the youngest of the third generation, at 28, to be affected, screening for the family was offered.

My grandmother (father's mother) must have been the carrier for the Lynch syndrome MLH1 gene mutation – we know this because her younger sister has the gene and had bowel cancer at age 42.

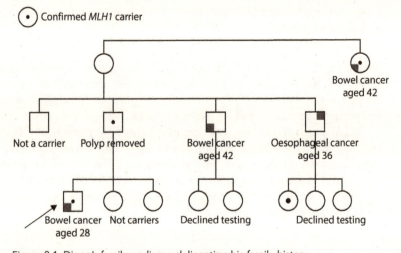

Figure 2.1 Dirren's family pedigree delineating his family history.

My grandmother had four sons:

- Son #1 – not a carrier.
- Son #2 – (my dad) carrier for the gene, but so far is dormant. He did require a small operation to remove a small section of bowel due to a large polyp. Both my sisters have been tested and neither is a carrier.
- Son #3 – carrier for Lynch and diagnosed with bowel cancer in 2014 age 52. He has two daughters who have declined the tests.
- Son #4 – carrier for the gene and died in 2000 aged 36 from oesophageal cancer – not tested but a confirmed carrier as his eldest daughter has the gene. She is one of three girls, but the only one in this family to be tested, the other two have decided not to know.

So, what did a diagnosis of Lynch syndrome mean for me? To know you have a 'genetic' condition, whether right or wrong when you say it out loud, it makes you instantly think 'something is wrong with me'. I had always felt fine and thought I was 'normal'. For a time I felt inferior, broken and different. However, those feelings soon disappeared as I focused on my physical recovery. From a medical point of view, in simple terms, it meant that the remaining part of my bowel and rectum were at high risk of cancer returning, especially as it had already hit me at such a young age.

A year after my initial diagnosis, I had my one-year check-up at St George's hospital. Who should I see when the curtain was pulled back but Gareth (Anisha's husband, whom I knew well)! After a moment of shock, I remember Gareth telling me I was next on his list and if I was ok with that? I'll never forget his exact wording: 'Once you have seen one bum hole, you've seen them all.' I wonder if he knows just how many he's seen? It made me laugh and put me at ease.

The colonoscopy felt fine, but there was a large polyp identified and it seemed inevitable that the cancer was going to come back. The best option now was to remove the remaining half of my existing colon and have a full colectomy.

It was at this point that my mindset wavered for the first time. I didn't want a stoma, I felt I was too young for a stoma and I knew if I had one it would be not reversible. The surgeon told me it was going to be 50/50 and I wouldn't know until I woke up from theatre whether I would have one.

Waiting for the op was an awful three months, because I made it that way. I kept watching videos and reading about stomas and people who were living lives without a large intestine. I went on a food marathon one month before my operation because I'd been told I would have to avoid certain foods with a stoma. I went to all my favourite restaurants and ate everything in large quantities. I put on twenty pounds but I didn't care, I had convinced myself that I was going to be on a plain diet for the rest of my life – so I might as well enjoy it while I could!

I woke up from my operation frantically feeling around my stomach area. Had the surgeon been able to connect the small intestine to the rectum or had he had to create a stoma? I remember my wife taking my hand and saying, 'It's ok, you don't have a stoma.'

Since that day I have not looked back. Mentally, I was stronger than I had ever been before. This mental conviction allowed my physical recovery to begin immediately. Within a few hours of being awake post op, I walked up and down the hospital corridor. Within one week, I was walking up and down the street. Within one month I was walking 5 km and after ten weeks I was running 10 km.

When I look back, I am not sure it really sank in properly until we were ready to start thinking about having children. We were told there was a 50/50 chance of passing the gene on, with it being more prevalent in males. I was adamant we needed to go down the IVF/pre-implantation genetic diagnosis* route, but I was acutely aware that all the hard work, pain and sacrifice would be experienced by my wife, and so it was only fair that she made the decision of how we should

---

* The process of IVF is described in Chapter 13 in further detail. The embryos produced are checked for the MLH1 change and then only the embryos which do not carry the genetic change are implanted back into the mother.

progress. Luckily for me, she agreed and we've been blessed with two beautiful daughters conceived via IVF, allowing us to eliminate the MLH1 gene altogether and forever. A huge relief for us, and for my parents as well.

I'm now 39 and have been in remission for seven years and nine months. I'm happy and healthy. Yes, I have to go to the toilet more frequently, but I've got used to it and to be honest I never give it a moment's thought.

I live my life taking each day as it comes, I don't worry about when or if the cancer will return. I choose to look at the positives and surround myself with like-minded people who look forward not backwards. I believe that my positive mental attitude coupled with my amazing support network is what drives me to be better and do better every single day.

What is Lynch syndrome?

Lynch syndrome, previously known as HNPCC (hereditary non-polyposis colorectal cancer), is a genetic condition with autosomal dominant inheritance. This means there is a 50 per cent chance of children or siblings also having Lynch syndrome as the gene is passed down. Having Lynch syndrome increases the risk of developing CRC before you are 50 and, in females, endometrial (womb) cancer. There is also a slight increased risk of other cancers such as stomach, liver, small intestine, pancreatic, bile duct, kidney, ureteral, ovarian, brain and certain skin cancers.

A genetic mutation occurs in genes called mismatch repair genes – MLH, MSH2, MSH6, PMS2, and EPCAM. These genes normally protect you from getting certain cancers by repairing DNA, but mutations in these genes prevent them from working properly. All UK hospitals now test for this routinely in all colon and endometrial cancer cases.

Astonishingly currently 95 per cent of cases in the UK are undiagnosed. It is estimated that 200,000 people in UK have Lynch. This has implications not just for the individual but for family members as well who could get genetically tested, and if positive be placed on early surveillance schedules. For example, colorectal cancer screening would reduce your risk of dying from CRC by 72 per cent if you were known to have Lynch syndrome and were in the appropriate screening programme.

Management of Lynch syndrome

Guidance varies between countries and current UK guidance is outlined below.

• **Lifestyle advice:** patients should be given general lifestyle advice to reduce their risk of cancer.

- **Chemoprevention with aspirin:** daily aspirin use to reduce the risk of colorectal cancer by approximately 50 per cent – 150 mg a day is recommended if less than 70 kg weight and 300 mg if over 70 kg. Please check with your doctor to ensure this is suitable before starting aspirin.
- **Risk-reducing surgery:** to reduce your chance of developing a cancer, may include removal of bowel and, in women, removal of the ovaries and womb (total hysterectomy) from the age of 40, or after child bearing. HRT will be offered to those with no contraindications.
- **Screening and surveillance:**
  - **Colonoscopies:** (every 2 years from the age of 25–35 depending on the gene mutation) to allow early detection of CRC.
  - ***Heliobacter pylori*:** this bacteria doesn't often cause symptoms, but it increases the risk of ulcers and stomach cancer. A course of antibiotics can eradicate the *H. pylori* bacteria, and therefore reduce the risk of stomach cancer developing.
  - **Family testing:** cascade testing for at-risk individuals and reproductive advice regarding future children (as Dirren received).

Colonic polyposis syndromes

These syndromes include familial adenomatous polyps (FAP) and MUTYH-associated polyposis (MAP). They are rare and there are multiple genes that can cause polyps to develop if they are not working properly. Most are associated with an increased risk of CRC. Due to the specialist nature of these syndromes, and the complexities of diagnosis and management, if a polyposis syndrome is suspected, patients will be referred to a genetics centre or a polyposis centre. (Colonoscopies are recommended every two years between the ages of 25–35 depending on the gene mutation – to allow early detection of CRC.)

Please see the Useful Resources section at the end of the book for further help and support for genetic conditions and bowel cancer.

The gut microbiome – the godfather of the gut

What is the gut microbiome?

Living inside each and every one of us are trillions of micro-organisms – bacteria, viruses and fungi, for example, that collectively make up a microbiome. Different organs are made up of different organisms but the organ receiving the most attention in terms of research is the gut microbiome, or microbiota. The make-up of the gut microbiome will also vary from person to person.

The gut microbiome has a huge effect on the health of humans, including helping control our immune system, digestion of fibre, energy production, protection against infections and maintenance of brain health. There has been so much interest in this topic over recent years, and it is thought that it may have a role in many conditions such as obesity, acne, asthma, mental health, ADHD, possibly diabetes, inflammatory bowel disease, irritable bowel syndrome, eczema, cancer, and immune function.

We know we can promote a healthy and diverse microbiome influenced by dietary factors (see Appendix), exercising, not smoking, getting a good night's sleep regularly and reducing stress levels. It is thought that the gut microbiome also plays an important role in the development of CRC. It has a role in the progression of cancer as well as responses to systemic treatment. Different diets will have different effects on the gut microbiome which may be protective and anti-inflammatory, or pro inflammatory leading to the formation of CRC.

The gut microbiome can influence the response to chemotherapy in CRC patients, and the severity of side effects from treatment. Future clinical trials and research will focus on the gut microbiome in oncology, as well as using the knowledge of the gut microbiome to influence treatments and future treatments for the possible prevention of CRC and to help improve patients' outcomes.

Early onset colorectal cancer (EOCRC)

Early onset colorectal cancer has been an increasing problem over the last 50 years. The incidence of EOCRC will possibly increase by a startling 140 per cent by 2030. The exact cause is unknown but it may be due to factors like obesity, less physical activity and increased antibiotic use early on in childhood, all of which can affect immunity and the gut microbiome.

There are stark differences between EOCRC and late-onset colorectal cancer (LOCRC), which are highlighted below.

- Anatomically EOCRC are more likely to be in the left side of the colon or in the rectum, compared with LOCRC.
- Epidemiologically, African Americans are 20 per cent more likely to have EOCRC than white Americans.
- Family, genetics and hereditary conditions are associated with 30 per cent of EOCRC compared with approximately 15 per cent of LOCRC. Those with EOCRC under the age of 40 will be offered genetic testing for all Lynch syndrome and polyposis genes in the UK and other countries.

It is clear that a lot more research into the rise of EOCRC is needed to provide more answers and hopefully help identify those at risk earlier as well as tailoring treatment more effectively.

3

How will I be investigated for colorectal cancer?

There is a variety of investigations involved in diagnosing CRC, as well as assessing its stage. Not everyone will undergo all the tests listed here, but an overview of what each test does is outlined below.

If you develop symptoms of possible bowel cancer (as outlined in Chapter 1) your doctor may suggest undertaking blood and stool tests initially. Depending on the results, you may be offered further tests, including a camera examination into your bowel known as a colonoscopy, or a scan known as a CT colonography.

If tests result in a diagnosis of CRC being made, you will need to undergo further investigations, including a CT scan and/or MRI scan and/or a PET scan to help determine what treatment you may require. These tests are known as staging investigations.

Blood tests

Simple blood tests can be used to identify signs of anaemia, or low iron levels, which can be a marker of bowel disease or signify blood loss, including CRC.

What is FIT testing?

When reaching a diagnosis of CRC, one of the first investigations you may have is a stool test known as a FIT (faecal immunochemical test) test. This may be undertaken in primary care (at your doctor's surgery), or as part of the national bowel cancer screening programme (please see Chapter 21).

This test detects microscopic traces of blood in your stool which are so small in volume they are not usually visible to the naked eye. In some countries, people are also able to buy FIT tests over the counter or online.

If a FIT test is found to be positive, you will normally be referred to hospital for consideration for further testing, such as a colonoscopy, but remember a positive FIT test does not necessarily mean you have bowel cancer.

Cologuard

In the US, a cologuard test may be used instead of a FIT test, and often in screening. It detects DNA changes in cancer cells that may have been shed by the cancer, which then pass in the stool through the colon. It also can detect blood loss in the gut. Again, much like the FIT test, if this test is positive, you will go onto have further tests such as a colonoscopy.

Colonoscopy

A colonoscopy is a test to check inside your bowel/colon to try to ascertain what is causing symptoms, or to investigate a positive FIT test.

A strong laxative is given prior to the procedure (bowel preparation) to fully clear the colon of all residual stool, so that a good view of the bowel can be achieved at the time of the examination.

A colonoscope is a long, thin, flexible tube with a small camera and light at the tip, which is passed into your bottom (rectum) and around the colon. You may be offered a light sedative and a painkiller through an injection beforehand to make you more comfortable during the procedure. Many patients are able to undergo a colonoscopy without sedation, and instead opt to use an inhaled painkiller called Entonox, otherwise known as 'laughing gas'.

The specialist performing the colonoscopy will be able to visualize the lining of your bowel from the rectum all the way around your colon to your appendix. If anything looks suspicious or unusual, a biopsy will usually be taken. The biopsy will be sent to a pathologist for further analysis.

It is very important to follow the dietary advice and bowel preparation instructions carefully (both the pre-procedural dietary advice and medication instructions) so that the inside of the colon and rectum is as clean as it possibly can be for a successful procedure. This allows the most accurate and thorough inspection of the bowel and reduces the chances of any abnormalities being missed. You want to try to avoid needing a repeat procedure because the bowel preparation has not worked well enough for the specialist to see what is going on!

Tips: Preparing for a colonoscopy

The diet

- Avoid high-fibre foods such as popcorn, nuts, seeds, raw vegetables, sweetcorn, peas, fried foods and bran.
- Try also to avoid beetroot, red jelly or any food products which are red in colour and which might mimic blood.
- Adhere to the dietary advice given and the fasting period.

Bottom care

- Ensure you are near to a toilet once you start taking the laxative medication. DO NOT make any plans to go out! Once the laxative starts working, it takes a while to stop and the effects on your bowel can be unpredictable, more so if you have already undergone bowel surgery or have a pre-existing bowel condition.
- Wear loose fitting clothing to allow a quick manouevre on to the toilet!
- Use water wipes, a bidet or very soft toilet tissue to help avoid a burning bottom from the catharsis which can result from bowel preparation.
- Apply a barrier nappy rash cream, such as metanium or bepanthen, or use vaseline, but make sure your bottom is dry before applying, otherwise this can cause more irritation. If pain occurs around the bottom, dab clear and avoid wiping aggressively.

Bowel prep

- The bowel prep may taste unpleasant. Suggestions to make it more palatable include: mixing it with other drinks, refrigerating it, drinking it through a straw, having a 'chaser' to get rid of the taste, holding your nose, chewing gum after or sucking ice cubes. To be honest, I just went ahead and drank it!

Hydration

- Rehydrate constantly until the time you are required to be nil by mouth.
- Drinking plenty of water or dilute squash is perfectly adequate, but I have found Dioralyte or flat Lucozade drinks helpful in staving off the dehydration that can result from bowel preparation.

- If you feel dizzy, try drinking a dissolved stock cube or if really hungry, some sugar can be dissolved in water. If you are well hydrated, this usually staves off the hunger.

General advice

- Plan the journey to your appointment (you don't want to be caught short) and make arrangements for someone to take you home afterwards in case you require a sedative to be given for the procedure (you can easily ask them to 'stand down' if not required).
- Broad advice is to plan to take the 24 hours before and the 24 hours after a colonoscopy off from work.

CT colonography

Some patients are deemed either not fit enough, or have other factors which place them at higher risk, to have a colonoscopy, for example frail or elderly patients, those with multiple medical problems, and those on blood-thinning medications. In these cases, an alternative test called a CT virtual colonography (or CTVC) can be arranged. This is a special type of CT scan which is specifically designed to examine the bowel.

The scanner produces two- and three-dimensional images of the whole of the large bowel. During the procedure, a thin flexible tube is passed into your bottom through which gas is pumped to distend the bowel, allowing good views of the large bowel and rectum to be achieved. Bowel preparation is still required before the examination, but sedative and painkiller injections are not. Diagnostically, it is equivalent to a colonoscopy in detecting small polyps in the bowel measuring 5 mm or greater. The disadvantage of this investigation, however, is that it does not allow for taking biopsies or removing polyps, and some patients may still be required to undergo a subsequent endoscopy if an abnormality is identified.

CEA (carcinoembryonic antigen)

This is a chemical that is elevated in some patients with a diagnosis of CRC. It is not usually used to detect bowel cancer, but is more commonly used as a marker of response to treatment for CRC, or in the surveillance phase.

Staging Investigations

CT scan

'The polo mint', a CT scan (computerized tomography) is a donut-shaped scanner that takes a series of X-rays to build a three-dimensional image of your internal body structures. A CT scan is used to determine whether the CRC is contained within the bowel, or whether there is evidence of spread into other structures/organs. You may have an injection of dye into one of your veins when the scan is done. This dye is called 'contrast' and can help obtain better visualization of certain structures. The injection of dye often gives patients a sensation of warmth rushing throughout the body, and can cause you to feel as though you are wetting yourself – but please don't worry, you probably aren't! The scan usually lasts 10–20 minutes.

MRI scan

'The open-ended tunnel', magnetic resonance imaging (MRI) uses strong magnetic fields and radio waves to produce detailed images of the inside of the body. An MRI scan is routinely used in the staging of rectal cancer as it is able to examine in great detail the structures that sit deep within the pelvis (including the rectum) which are not usually well seen on CT scans. The information provided by the MRI scan will help determine what treatment for rectal cancer will be offered. It is a painless procedure that can take between 15 and 90 minutes to complete, depending on the body area(s) being scanned. It is extremely noisy in the scanner, but you will be given headphones through which relaxing music or sounds are usually played, so try not to be alarmed. Contrast dye may also need to be used, and side effects include dizziness, headache, a skin rash or nausea.

MRI scans can be a very daunting prospect for those with claustrophobia (which I suffer to a reasonable degree). However, I have managed to overcome my fears of MRI scanning with some therapy and desensitization work. There are also open-air scanners, but unfortunately these are not widely available. Referral to one of these scanners may result in a delay to the scan being performed, but you should make enquiries if you suffer from claustrophobia. If you have significant anxiety about the MRI, your GP may be able to prescribe you a dose of sedation to take prior to the scan, which I have been asked to do on many occasions in my role as a GP, and which I have also found beneficial in calming my own nerves before my scans. Remember that if you do take a sedative, you will need to be accompanied both to and from the appointment.

PET scan

Positron emission tomography (PET) scans involve injecting a radioactive sugar (FDG) into the blood, which mainly collects in cancer cells. This will produce images of inside the body and highlight any hot spots where cancer cells may have migrated. They are not routinely performed in all bowel cancer patients. They are helpful for investigating confirmed cases of cancer and can determine how far the cancer has spread and how the cancer is responding to treatment. PET scans are often combined with CT scans or MRI scans to produce even more detailed images.

Waiting for results

I have profound empathy with those who reach out to me after a cancer diagnosis, as I fully appreciate that the waiting (be it for scans, biopsy results, multidisciplinary team outcomes, or hospital appointments) is the most agonizing time of any cancer diagnosis. The uncertainty about what lies ahead, and the lack of a plan in the early stages, can induce levels of anxiety which are physically debilitating, psychologically damaging, and which can render the most highly functioning individuals absolutely helpless. I will talk about this more later in Chapter 14.

So, you've had all your tests. What next?

The multidisciplinary team meeting

After you have had all the necessary investigations, your results will be discussed in the multidisciplinary team (MDT) meeting. The MDT meeting usually comprises a surgeon, a pathologist, an oncologist, a radiologist and a cancer specialist nurse. This team convenes on a weekly basis and comes to a collective decision regarding the stage and grade of the cancer, and this in turn determines the most appropriate management plan for your individual case, taking into account the most up-to-date evidence regarding treatments currently available. Sometimes the MDT meeting may determine that further tests are needed before a decision regarding treatment can be made. Try not to be disappointed if this should occur – they are trying to make the best decision for you, and may simply need more information to facilitate this.

Further MDT discussion will also take place after any surgery performed, to discuss the final cancer grading and staging. These may change after the removed tumour has been examined by a pathologist, as they are able to provide a more detailed examination of the cancer and its relationship to the bowel wall and nearby lymph nodes than the pre-operative staging tests can provide.

What are the stages of bowel cancer?

The stage of cancer describes its size and whether it has spread. To determine the stage, we require tests, including scans and tissue samples from surgery or a biopsy.

For colorectal cancer, the TNM staging system is most commonly used:

T – describes how far the tumour has grown into the wall of the bowel.

N – describes whether the cancer has spread to lymph nodes.

M – describes if the cancer has spread to another site in the body, commonly the lung and liver with regard to colorectal cancer but it can spread to other body parts (secondary or metastatic colorectal cancer).

Understanding the cancer

The bowel wall contains various layers (see Figure 3.1 below).

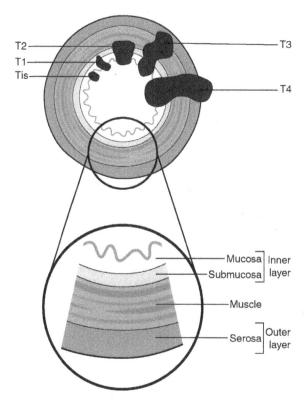

Figure 3.1 TNM number staging

This image was produced by Macmillan Cancer Support and is reused with permission.
Additional labels have been used.

Tis – tumour has grown into the mucosa only – this is the earliest stage and is also known as 'in situ'	
T1	Tumour is in the inner layer of the bowel called the submucosa (inner lining).
T2	Tumour has grown into the muscle layer of the bowel wall.
T3	Tumour has grown through the muscle and into the outer layer of the bowel wall called the serosa, but has not gone through it.
T4	Can be split into two stages, T4a and T4b. Tumour has grown through the outer layer of the bowel wall (serosa) and through the peritoneum (the membrane surrounding the outside of the bowel wall).
T4a	Tumour has caused a hole in the bowel wall (perforation) and the cancer cells have spread outside the bowel.
T4b	Tumour or other parts of the bowel have grown into nearby organs.

N – Nodes	
N0	No lymph nodes contain cancer cells.
N1	Up to three lymph nodes nearby contain cancer cells.
N2	Four or more lymph nodes contain cancer cells.
M – Metastases	
M0	No cancer spread to distant organs.
M1	Cancer has spread to distant organs, for example lungs and liver.

All this information can then be used to give us a staging of the cancer.

- Stage 0 Tis N0M0 – earliest stage and cancer is only in mucosa.
- Stage 1 T1N0M0 or T2N0M0 – cancer has grown into the submucosa or muscle only but no spread elsewhere.
- Stage 2 T3N0M0 T4N0M0 – cancer has grown through the muscle wall or through outer layer of bowel wall but no spread to lymph nodes or elsewhere.
- Stage 3 any T N1M0 or any T N2M0 – cancer is any size but has spread to lymph nodes nearby but nowhere else (T3N1M0 was the stage of cancer I had).
- Stage 4 any T any N M1 – cancer is any size which may have spread to lymph nodes nearby. The cancer has now spread to a distant site such as the liver or lungs.

Knowing the cancer stage can help doctors as part of a multidisciplinary approach to determine treatment strategies. It can also give an estimate of life expectancy and statistical chance of cure.

Clinical trials testing new treatments for cancer tend to be stratified for specific cancer stages, to determine how effective the new treatment is. So staging is important in clinical research, too.

Grading

The pathologist will analyse the cells under the microscope once the tumour has been removed. This can give the grade of the tumour and may determine how quickly a tumour may develop, grow or spread.

The grade of the tumour describes how abnormal the tumour cells are under a microscope. Grades include:

- Grade 1 (low grade) – the cells are well differentiated and tend to look similar to normal cells. In general, these cancers are less likely to spread than higher grade cancers.
- Grade 2 (moderate grade) – cancer cells look more abnormal.
- Grade 3 (high grade) – the tumour cells are poorly differentiated and grow quicker as well as look more abnormal.

A cancer specialist nurse will usually contact patients after the MDT meeting has taken place to inform them of the outcome of the meeting and will arrange appointments with the most appropriate specialists. This is when you will hear what your proposed treatment plan will be, what your options are, and it will allow you the opportunity to ask any questions you may have. This is when you may feel a slight sense of relief from all the waiting, as you now can embark on the next phase of your cancer journey, perhaps getting you one step closer to removing or shrinking that tumour.

4

Sharing news with loved ones

My husband had the unenviable task of announcing to all family members the news that had rocked our world soon after my colonoscopy. I was in a state of shock and disbelief, and couldn't for the life of me think how I would impart this sort of information, knowing the devastation it would cause.

How someone decides to share their news (or not) is very individual. I very much felt I didn't want this to happen to anyone else, wanting everyone to get over the shock of it all at the same time. This was in the hope that they would be ready to have all hands on deck for the hurdles that would follow, without having to explain again and again the devastation, like a plaster being ripped off multiple times from the same deep wound.

Some may feel that they need to protect their loved ones from the emotional burden of cancer – especially parents, for example. I can't imagine what it is like as a parent to see your child (no matter how old) be diagnosed with a life-threatening illness and then proceed through all manner of treatment. I felt the need to protect my mum, so I would often organize others – such as my parents-in law, or my brothers – to look after me or the children during my darkest times, as I couldn't bear for her to see me like that, or cause her any more distress or worry than she was probably already feeling. I'm sure she would feel differently reading this but, at the time, I chose what I thought was best for all those involved, including myself, as there were times I needed just to exist without worrying about anyone else.

Below are some tips on how to break the news to loved ones and things to think about; not all of these will be right for you and yours.

Tips: Breaking the news to loved ones

- Do what's right for you. You may choose to tell your partner and no one else, you may choose to broadcast it. There is no right or wrong. The way you handle sharing this news is all part of the way you are coping with cancer and is an active coping mechanism.
- Prepare what you want to say and how much you want to share. Be honest.
- Think about how to disseminate information so you're not repeating yourself multiple times, whether this is by WhatsApp, social media, email, or even letter. Conversely, ask others to help you make phone calls and arm them with the correct information.
- Think of a sentence starter, for example, 'You know I haven't been feeling well recently? Well, tests have shown ...'
- Ask what they already know and understand from the situation and give important information in bitesize pieces.
- Silence – this is ok, and non-verbal communication such as hugging and crying is just as important. Ask them: what they are thinking.
- Be prepared for a whole host of reactions (I'll share more on this below).
- Share your worries and thoughts.
- Finally accept support offered and don't forget to ask if not volunteered. They will be in a state of shock too.

Sharing news with children

Looking back, this was without doubt one of the trickiest moments in my life, knowing that I was about to share information that they might not fully understand the significance of, but which undoubtedly would cause pain and heartache for all.

How you impart this information will depend on your child, their understanding and experience of illness or cancer in the past, as well as their age. You know them best. There is no right or wrong time to tell them, although it's important to be honest as you can. If you don't have all the answers, that's absolutely fine, but it is important to tell them this. Some people choose to tell their children when they have a plan of action following all the results, to help ease that fear of the unknown.

We decided to tell our children the day after I was diagnosed. K and S knew something was wrong the moment we arrived back from hospital, and although as a parent your first instinct is to protect them, withholding this information when they are aware the atmosphere has changed can leave them feeling vulnerable. Phone calls were being made, my mum had suddenly turned up out of the blue, people were coming and going from the house, tears at the doorstep, flowers being left. It didn't leave much to the imagination. Trying to explain this to the children when the reality had not sunk in, the diagnosis unprocessed, the situation incomprehensible, was near impossible.

I can't actually remember how my children, aged six and seven, responded that particular day, The next day we were due to visit my brother-in-law for his 40th birthday. Apologies, D, not exactly how I would have wanted to wish you happy birthday – in my sleep-deprived, distracted state, our trip was in a bid to maintain as much normality as possible. As the front door opened, my daughter blurted out, 'Mummy has cancer' and then skipped off! We looked at each other bemused, my family in shock, but I knew this was S just processing the information given and also gauging an adult's reaction to the remark. What I realized over time was there were many more questions to follow, including, 'Mummy, will you die?' A question that no one wants to hear, but in this situation, we had to face up to. Other questions included, 'Can I get cancer?' and 'Daddy, you remove bowel cancers, why can't you remove Mummy's?' At which point high-tech diagrams were drawn of polyps and early bowel cancers, along with video footage of endoscopies. This took their interest to another level, but I guess they are the children of medics, after all.

I've met parents who ask my advice, as a GP, about how to tell the children about cancer. Sometimes they don't want to tell their children. Because they are scared. Because they want to protect them. Because they don't know how to. Because they are worried about their reaction. What I discuss with parents is this. Being honest with them signals to the child that you trust them, that you are in this boat together. That you are a team. Together you will get to the finish line, whenever and whatever that may be. It will make them feel less anxious and give them the space to ask questions and verbalize how they feel. Doing this can reduce their fear and anxiety. I know from personal experience that it can also bring you closer as a unit, whereby you are all supporting each other. And although this surely tested their resilience, this experience has taught my children so much more and is now a part of their tapestry.

My expert psychotherapist, Danni, knows only too well the long-term implications for children if parents aren't honest about a cancer diagnosis. For example, she explains how they can develop trust issues. It is by no means an easy conversation to have, but in the long run, you will be protecting your child(ren) and preserving your relationship with them. Not being honest may lead to fear and anxiety, as they will be aware something is wrong. They might build up ideas in their head about situations which may be unfounded – in the face of lots of whispering and maybe tears, a child is perhaps far more likely to think that 'mummy and daddy are getting divorced' rather than the reality of 'mummy has cancer'.

It is also important to remember that little people have very big ears, and there have been instances when people have been discussing their cancer diagnosis with friends, or others have been chatting among themselves, and a child has overheard. In addition, the Chinese whispers that occur in the playground may reach a child who is unaware of their parent's diagnosis, which can be devastating for the child. It is best they hear this from you as the parent.

We've come together to offer this list of tips for you to think about when telling children your news.

Tips: Telling children about a cancer diagnosis

- Prepare what you are going to say at this stage. You may find that writing down what you would like to discuss helps align your thoughts. Ensure you have spoken to your medical team so you are armed with facts, and they may be able to signpost you to resources to help support the children. Avoid too much detail as it may be overwhelming, but do explain words such as 'chemotherapy' and 'radiotherapy'.
- Plan to tell them in a place where they feel comfortable and safe.
- Use open-ended questions, for example, 'What do you know about cancer?', and share experiences of others they may be able to relate to.
- Try to use the word 'cancer' or 'bad cells' rather than 'poorly' or 'ill'. They may associate cancer with anyone who is feeling 'poorly' or 'ill' in the future. Generally speaking, Danni advises that those

of primary school age (five and above) may be able to understand the word cancer depending on their maturity but if not, or younger, Danni suggests using the words 'bad cells' and 'good cells'.

- Prepare yourself for their reaction. Some children may look at you and then immediately ask 'What's for tea?' as if they haven't heard, others may cry or look confused. Whatever it is, be prepared that it might not be the reaction you were expecting. However, give them the time and space to process.
- Check their understanding of what's going on and allow them to direct the conversation with their reactions and thoughts.
- Keep terminology simple and keep to the point, not dwelling too much on the future and the 'what ifs'.
- Tell all the children in the house together so no one is left feeling the burden or left out. Occasionally parents think it is best to tell the older children and hide it from the younger child, but this is quite a weight for one child to carry and it can unintentionally break trust with the other child.
- Tell them as a family, and if you are a single-parent family, consider support from another family member or friend. Sometimes the person affected by cancer doesn't want to be there, and that's ok, as long as they know what is being said.
- Use visual aids, books or websites (see Useful Resources section).
- Explain how things may be different moving forwards while you undergo treatment.
- You don't have to tell them everything at once if you feel it will be overwhelming, but do check their understanding and what they have heard and absorbed. You may find you need to repeat information, especially if they are younger.
- Allow space and time for questions with an open door policy if they have any concerns.
- Talking to children at regular intervals keeps them from fearing the worst and avoids them feeling isolated from the family and situation.
- Let them know not all cancers are the same and each person, even if they do have a similar cancer, will have a different experience.
- Inform the school so they can keep an eye out for them and ensure support is available.
- And finally, remind them they are totally loved.

When you have told them, it is important to address their concerns and questions as honestly as you can. If they feel you aren't addressing their concerns, they may become fearful that you are hiding something and lose trust.

I often found cancer-related questions would pop up at the most unusual and peculiar moments, highlighting the fact that their little minds were always processing. It's paramount they understand they cannot catch cancer, it's no one's fault, they will always be looked after, and they are free to talk about it at any time.

Also don't be surprised if they become more withdrawn, their behaviour changes or they become more attached to the other parent or family member. This is quite normal, although I appreciate this can be heartbreaking too.

I was so fortunate to have access to a children's counsellor at the holistic cancer centre attached to the hospital I received treatment in. The Fountain Centre were phenomenal at facilitating difficult conversations, both with and without us present, through play therapy. I actually found it fascinating the way they used toys and play to explain not only cancer and its treatment, but the emotions and everything that comes with it. I informed the children's school of my diagnosis and they offered support and a 'safe' space outside of their home, as home may not be their 'safe' place (temporarily) anymore. They forged a strong bond with their ELSA (emotional learning support assistant) at school, and found their weekly sessions with her invaluable.

And, as adults do, children can also display phases of grief which manifest through changes in behaviour. We found this happened more so after treatment finished, when they felt they could breathe and to them, there was no longer a need to tiptoe around me. However, we all had a period of adjustment to try to embrace, and live with, the 'new normal' gauntlet that cancer had thrown down.

If you're ever worried or concerned that your child is struggling, please do go and see your GP or family doctor and ask for help. Professional counselling may be helpful too. There are plenty of books out there, but unfortunately, I never quite found the right one for my children despite scouring the internet. S definitely experienced quite a severe sleep anxiety and separation anxiety (specifically with me) after treatment, which has taken a long time to recover from, requiring some professional help.

When speaking to teenagers about cancer, the understanding and outlook may be different. Teenagers may have been taught about cancer at school or may have had friends who have experienced cancer in their family. Teenagers and older children may not want to talk about things as much, as they do not want to be seen as different by their peers. However, the principles of discussing a diagnosis above still apply and they should know that there is help and support if they need it. Riprap, Hope Support Services and Macmillan Cancer Centres have resources for teenagers who have a parent with cancer that you can access.

Carpe diem

Remember that children will usually bounce back and be ok with love, honesty and a robust support system. Children and young people live in the moment more than adults so, as much as you can, if you try to live in the moment too, this will help them cope with their parent having cancer.

Finally, you know your child better than anyone so be led by them and most definitely, listen to your gut.

Managing people's reactions

You have made the brave step of disseminating the 'I have cancer' news. You will be absolutely amazed at the spectrum of responses you'll receive once you tell people you have cancer and throughout your treatment. I've heard it all, from 'It was God's will' to 'Maybe try some papaya?'. Nothing surprised me, but I appreciate it wasn't always easy to manage.

From the people who rush round offering bundles of love, care and attention to those who avoid you on the street when you walk past.

From those who go into 'practical military operation' mode to those who come crying on your doorstep.

From those who are practical and hands on, organizing your logistics, to those who ghost you and walk away.

From those who come out of the woodwork, to those who crawl back in.

From the hushed whispers to those who treat you like china.

From those who say, 'Let me know what I can do', to those who just get on and do it.

Be prepared for the good, the bad and the ugly.

Whatever the reaction, it is important to give people time to absorb the information you have given them, process this and overcome their own shock they may feel. The ripple effect of a cancer diagnosis is so huge, and one that I appreciate so much more as a doctor now, in my day-to-day practice. The confusion, fear and helplessness that people can experience themselves once the news filters through can be crippling. It can also trigger emotions they've experienced when other loved ones around them have had a diagnosis themselves. Eventually, once their own feelings are processed, most people will be falling over themselves to be supportive.

Below are some of the reactions you might encounter after diagnosis and through treatment, many of which I encountered too.

Distress – 'How will we get through this? I'm so distraught'

This is totally understandable. The word 'cancer' can launch a grenade of fear at many people when mentioned. There were plenty of times shortly after diagnosis when people would turn up on my doorstep in tears. My husband, I know, found this incredibly frustrating and unhelpful, but he himself was in practical military operation mode, shedding tears with friends around me at times, but rarely with me. I imagine G felt he had to be strong to see me through this. Me? Well, I was still feeling numb, so when people cried in front of me I didn't mind. I thought it was a natural process and I would probably have been the same, had I been in their shoes. Maybe it was the doctor in me, ever ready to listen to the upset and hurt people experience in life. I felt people were with me in my sadness and understood the upheaval this situation would cause. Through treatment, I also cried with friends, which in itself was incredibly cathartic. Being told not to cry? I don't think that's beneficial, the bucket of tears needs to be emptied now and again, and I encourage people to set themselves time to have an unfiltered cry.

I think we should be mindful to try not to blame individuals for their own distress. At the end of the day, they love you and are scared, and shocked. It's because they love you or it's triggered an experience(s) they've had themselves. If indeed you do find other people's distress upsetting, do remind them gently that you, too, are dealing with the distress and actually haven't got the capacity currently to deal with anyone else's as well.

Toxic positivity – 'I'm sure you will be fine'

Toxic positivity is the belief that no matter how dire or difficult a situation is, people should maintain a positive mindset constantly.

Often unintentionally, people can dismiss distress and the negative way someone may be feeling, responding with false reassurance, rather than with empathy, validation, support and compassion. Expert opinions suggest that toxic positivity can be damaging for an individual's mental health.

For example, when someone says 'positive vibes only', this can be quite unintentionally upsetting when every day that person might be going through hell, feeling utterly rubbish, and all they want to do is curl up in a ball. It can be exhausting (and totally normal) to have days when you don't feel upbeat or positive, even though your outlook to undergoing treatment is positive. It is so important to acknowledge the pain, the fear and the anxiety and be honest if you are unsure what to say.

I have heard it all through cancer treatment and beyond. Most of the time, I would shut it out. Deep down, I knew that such comments originated from a meaningful place but when it happened time and time again, it could really grind, causing more harm or upset than good.

Here are some examples of what can be said, and how it could be worded differently to have a more positive impact on the recipient.

Toxic positivity	Try saying this instead
It could be worse.	I know things are really hard right now but I'm here for you.
It will all be fine.	How are you feeling? This must be so tough.
Be positive. Stay positive. Positive vibes only.	I'm here for you through the good and the bad. I'm not going anywhere.
Keep fighting and don't give up!	I can see you're stressed/struggling, could I do the food shop for you/help at all?
Everything happens for a reason.	Do you want to talk about it?

See the good in everything.	It's probably really hard to see any good in this situation, but one day at a time right now.
I did it, so can you!	It's ok if you are struggling. We are all different, and have different situations, dealing with different things in different ways.
None of us knows how long we've got, I could get run over by a bus tomorrow.	It must be really scary living with this uncertainty.

Sometimes we can force the pressure of positivity on ourselves, which in turn can also be harmful to our mental health, when sometimes it's ok not to be ok. All emotions are allowed. If you know someone with cancer, ensure you listen and validate their feelings. Offer support.

I found the best way of managing it was to just let it pass over my head. Or laugh about it! As I say, people are often trying to say what they think will be supportive and caring, but out of ignorance or fear they say something nonsensical instead. Remember, they may not fully comprehend the potential hurt or uselessness of such comments unless they have trodden a similar path at some point, but you do need your army. So, if you can, be patient and let it all just wash over you, or gently point out how it can make you feel.

Fad diets and misinformation – 'I'm trying to give you some helpful advice'

We all have been offered something that is not conventional with regard to helping with cancer. However, it can be confusing or, frankly, harmful when you're presented with such information. This is even more so when targeted at vulnerable groups like patients with cancer, those in search of hope, or those with low self-esteem or self-confidence who are just so desperate to be 'cured'.

There is a plethora of misinformation online. Try to avoid this at all costs unless there is an evidence base, and if you're unsure, please check with your specialist. There were situations where people close to me, with an eagerness to help, would suggest a variety of diets – all from a good place, but actually not helpful at all. I was offered papaya, turmeric, alkaline diets, and a variety of other 'remedies' that simply weren't going to help treat my cancer. Some of these fads and diets are, quite frankly, dangerous; for example the alkaline diet could potentially see you ending up malnourished, deficient in iron, calcium, zinc, vitamin B12, and vitamin D! (A systematic review has shown there is a lack of evidence to show this diet cures or prevents cancer, in case you were wondering.)

I am often asked about, and offered, various 'alternative therapies' which have no evidence base or scientific data to support their use. I have no problem using complementary therapies – I was brought up by parents who owned a health food shop for most of their lives, and alternative medicines and complementary medicines were staples. However, if you do want to trial any of these approaches, look at the available literature and discuss them your specialist or oncologist. For example, my mum insisted I tried CBD oil to help with pain and sleep in the depths of chemo, and after consulting my oncologist, I did indeed take it with some success. However, this was alongside treatment.

Be careful and, if you're unsure, ask your specialist before experimenting.

Limelight – 'That parent with cancer'

Honestly, having cancer does give you a new-found status. One that I would totally give back in a heartbeat. Overnight, it sets you apart from everyone else. Yet I still looked like me at the beginning. Alas, the school run becomes an obstacle course of well-meaning but some-times awkward pleasantries you'd rather avoid, because you have become 'that mum with cancer', 'the doctor with cancer', and you feel your true identity initially drift and then progressively ebb away. People either walk away or rush towards you.

There is little you can do about the sometimes-unwanted atten-tion. On the days I was bedridden on chemo, others would walk my children to school. On the days I could walk them there, I simply couldn't face anyone. I would use an alternative back way to get to school with less traffic and fewer people and less interaction, purely for my self-preservation. Social anxiety became real, chemo stripping me of my extrovert streak, albeit temporarily.

It is difficult to escape, but with time, rest assured that it does (eventually) become old news and the attention fades once more, almost as quickly as it came.

Ghosting – 'Now you see me, now you don't'

Some people run a mile. Some people hide. They can't cope and don't know what to say or do.

Ghosting describes the practice of ending all communication and contact with another person without any warning, and ignoring all subsequent attempts at reconciliation. Often, it is a symptom of their not being able to cope with what you are going through. Calling that person if you wanted to, to try to put them at ease, is an option. If you are faced with someone you know receiving a diagnosis, saying nothing really shouldn't be an option. If you don't know what to say, it is fine to admit it, as this in itself will facilitate a conversation, even if it feels awkward and unnerving to begin with. 'Cancer ghosting' also refers to people you thought would be there for you but aren't or can't for whatever reason, which can be tremendously disappointing. We also know that cancer is often taboo in certain communities such as ethnic minority groups, when individuals might be ousted from the community when diagnosed, something I will talk about more later.

I've – painfully – been a victim of cancer ghosting. It's not uncommon, as I've subsequently found when discussing my own difficulties with others. It sucked an awful lot of my energy during my treatment.

In hindsight, I wish I had not wasted as much energy on these situations. Individuals' reactions were more of a reflection on themselves rather than indicating anything wrong with me. What I struggled with most was how anyone would treat me in such a way at probably the lowest point in my life, when I knew I would have tried to move heaven and earth if the boot had been on the other foot. Alas, after much therapy, time and conversations, I've tried to find a way forward, and I have had to lay some of these ghosts to rest so as not to waste any more precious time. After all, life is too short.

You have my utter sympathy if this has happened to you.

Fussing – 'Will you just stop fussing?'

'Do you need an extra pillow? You need to eat more. You need to sleep more. You need to get some fresh air. Do you need me to blow your nose, or even wipe your bum?'

It all comes from the heart, some people need to feel useful as a method of coping, but it can feel overwhelming, suffocating and overbearing, when all you want is some peace and quiet.

Do communicate this, gently, to the wonderful soul who is merely trying to help. For example, 'What I need right now is rest, and actually for you to rest, but I'll call you if I need you.'

'How can I help?'

I was often asked this question during treatment and subsequently afterwards by friends who had had loved ones diagnosed, asking me, 'What did you find most helpful?'

I was lucky to have the most supportive network that I renamed my Dream Team. They set up a group that I could text to ask for help, support, or just to rant at, especially on the dark days or when I was in hospital alone.

I was asked by my friends, 'What do you need?' I actually didn't know, but as time went on, I knew I wanted to maintain as much normality as possible, especially for the children. I'm a food lover and very particular about making food from scratch and eating healthy, well-balanced meals. (Though don't get me wrong, I love a takeaway and eating out as much as the next person.) In the blink of an eye, my friends had organized an amazing weekday rota. So when we didn't have family staying to help, mouthwatering dishes or pre-prepared bought meals were delivered daily to our door.

Childcare was the other massive headache. Throughout the whole time I was in treatment, G was only allowed one week of carer's leave to help. He worked long hours, out of the house by 7 a.m. and back after 7 p.m. if not later most days. It was going to be a logistical nightmare and I was really worried. So again, my friends and family stepped up, formulating childcare rotas so the children didn't miss out, even if they were pushed from pillar to post some days, something I'm sad they had to endure but with, I'm sure, no lasting effects.

Tips: How to offer help and support

- Listen – the ability to sit and listen to someone who has been diagnosed with cancer is the single most important thing anyone can do. Let them talk, without any judgement. This makes them feel seen, less alone, and to have their feelings validated. Acknowledge their feelings and do your best not to invalidate them by sweeping over concerns.
- Try to avoid giving unsolicited advice unless it is asked for.
- Educate yourself about the illness and treatment – this stops unnecessary confusion and fear, and prevents lots of questions being fired at the patient when they are already exhausted and vulnerable. Cancer charity websites have an abundance of literature.
- Be receptive and supportive of treatment decisions and choices the cancer patient makes. As a doctor, I've seen many situations where family members feel the patients should be considering alternative treatment options or are disappointed that the treatment offered may have been declined due to a multitude of reasons. Either way, if a patient has capacity, and they have all the information available to them regarding treatment, it is their wish and however frustrating or upsetting this may be, it has to be respected.
- Offer practical help and form a group with others (food rota, lifts to and from hospital and accompanying to appointments, hospital visits, childcare, dog walks, shopping).
- Offer to go out for a coffee, a walk, a trip to the garden centre, anything that the person before cancer was interested in or which might give them a change of scene.
- Stay connected – text, cards, email, Zoom calls, FaceTime, visits. Whatever that person needs, and don't forget that this connection needs to continue beyond diagnosis, through treatment and for some time AFTER cancer.
- Remember the person before cancer and try to keep normality as much as you can for them and their family. Sometimes this may include the patient wanting to carry on tasks that you could help with to keep normality for themselves like cooking and cleaning.
- Don't forget the caregiver. Check in, offer them some respite, some fun of their own. Behind the scenes, they are working tirelessly – my husband not only with his day job, but keeping everything going at home, with me and with the children, when he could.
- Be prepared that your loved one will not return to 'normal' immediately after treatment ends, emotionally or physically. Be aware that this is just the beginning of their 'new normal', a concept we will talk about later on. Needless to say, this is when the processing starts for patients so please keep the support going. They will find it much more difficult to ask when treatment ends.

5

It's treatment time

The A team

Before we move on to treatment types, let's take a look at your A Team. The health professionals who will help you through treatment, trying to preserve as much quality of life as possible, keeping you on the straight and narrow as much as they can.

I mentioned the multidisciplinary team earlier – the people involved in your care including your surgeon, oncologists, radiologist and pathologist. There are, additionally, numerous other health professionals you may encounter through your cancer experience. These angels will guide you through the wilderness, playing their role to optimize your care, so do tap into their knowledge. Ask questions. Take a second pair of ears, or take notes at each encounter.

Let me introduce your team.

Clinical cancer nurse specialist (CNS)

The oracle. The person who co-ordinates and personalizes your care and your first port of call for many issues, during and after treatment, if there is an issue related to bowel cancer. They orchestrate the multidisciplinary team meetings and provide in-depth knowledge about colorectal cancer, as well as offering support, and assessing holistic needs.

My follow-ups, scans, and colonoscopies are all arranged by my legend of a CNS, Angie. She also rings with all my results. If I have a problem – new symptoms that I'm worried about related to post-operative or treatment issues, or worse, a potential symptom of recurrence – I would contact my CNS, and have done so. You can also contact your GP or family doctor if you don't feel you have this support available, and I often see patients for this reason.

I am very fortunate to have a cancer nurse who has really supported me; she listens to me, always manages to alleviate my anxieties and can read me like a book. Angie had worked with my husband previously too and so she understood the unique challenges of being both patient and medic.

Oncology specialist nurse

There is usually an oncology treatment hotline manned by a specialist oncology nurse, so if you run into any difficulties with chemotherapy, this is your lifeline. Difficulties could include side effects of chemotherapy, signs of infection or fever, or a question relating to medication, for example. I remember tapping into them one night as I believed I had developed a stomach bug. Their advice was superb, and clear instructions given in case of any eventuality, so make sure you have their number on speed dial!

Stoma specialist nurse

The stoma nurse will provide information pre- and post-formation of the stoma, they will site the stoma and provide education and support on the management of a stoma physically and mentally. They come to see you on the ward after your stoma has been placed, and teach you how to manage and change your stoma. They were such a godsend when I had a few nights with various stoma problems, and they always knew what to do when I phoned them the next day, explaining terms like 'pancaking' (see Chapter 6).

Oncology dietician

Oh what to eat? It really did feel like this some days, but cancer specialist dieticians really helped me manage my difficulties with a change in diet following my stoma. They understood my desire to have a high-fibre diet as I always had previously, but many of these foods didn't agree with the stoma! So they gave me ideas to help with this. They also helped with my lack of appetite during chemotherapy and taught me how best to manage this. They can help anyone feeling nauseous, having issues with constipation or diarrhoea, finding it difficult to keep weight on, or eating through treatment. Oncology dieticians can help ensure you have good nutrition (sometimes with the help of supplements) and stay hydrated, which can help with quality of life.

Pharmacist

Specialized oncology pharmacists help patients manage a concoction of new drug therapies, optimizing their action and trying to minimize toxicity. They can answer queries related to your medication. Community pharmacists can also help with general medication queries.

Holistic cancer centre

In the UK, there is a variety of centres, for example those run by Macmillan and Maggie's, Penny Brohn UK, as well as many others. They are a hub of support services for those diagnosed with cancer, full of a range of alternative therapists, mental health support, counselling, and support for family members or carers.

The Fountain Centre is a charity-run holistic centre attached to the hospital I received treatment in (Royal Surrey NHS Foundation Trust), so my family and I were very fortunate that this was on the doorstep of treatment. This was one of the most important places for my family and me as we clambered on board the cancer train. I've already mentioned how the children received counselling and play therapy from this unit, and I spent at least 15 months receiving counselling from their service, from Danni (the psychotherapist sharing her invaluable input into this book as well). I also undertook a variety of alternative therapies there, including acupuncture for sciatica and peripheral neuropathy, reflexology and hypnotherapy for panic attacks early on. The therapists were incredible, and even came to the ward.

Research nurse/doctor

If you are asked to be part of a trial, you may be seen by a research doctor or nurse. They will be asking you questions to ensure you are eligible for their study and will then take you through the ins and outs of what may be involved. I participated in two trials and was very keen to help.

Physiotherapist

A physiotherapist can not only help with any mobility issues post-surgery, they can also help improve strength and endurance, and studies show they can improve quality of life measures in cancer patients. They can also help with pelvic floor health, essential for bowel control.

In addition to the people and organizations above, there is a whole host of other health professionals who might make up your team. Lean on them, let them support you, inform you and help you through cancer and beyond.

Questions?

As you read this book, you may have many questions. Some I will answer later in the book, some will be specific to your own cancer. Below, I have made short, non-exhaustive lists of questions to think about asking your specialist team, with space to add your own.

I know when I was going through this process, my mind was often numb, and I had my husband advocating for me, so at times I almost switched off and trusted the process, especially in the early days. Keeping a list of questions before you see your specialist can ensure you have all the answers, rather than walking out of the room and thinking, 'Oh, I forgot to ask...' More and more, we are seeing patients advocate for themselves, which can be an extremely helpful tool, empowering them to feel more in control when embarking on life-changing and disruptive treatment.

Questions to ask your surgeon

- What surgery do I need, and why?
- How advanced is the cancer?
- What are the complications or side effects of surgery?
- How risky is the procedure?
- How will going to the toilet for a poo be affected?
- Are there any alternative options?
- How long will I be in hospital for?
- How long will recovery take?
- Will I need a stoma? Will it be permanent?
- What will the scars be like?
- Is the surgery keyhole (laparoscopic), open or robotic? If you are unable to do the surgery I'm hoping for, do you know someone who could facilitate this or where I could have it done?
- When can I go back to work, or drive?

51

Questions to ask your oncologist

Oncology is the study of cancer and an oncologist will help diagnose, assess and decide the best treatment as part of a multidisciplinary team. Their aim is to provide the best possible outcome for the patient, whether that be curing the cancer or offering palliative care.

Below are some questions that you may want to ask your oncologist about cancer treatment, be it chemotherapy, radiotherapy or immunotherapy or target therapy.

- What are the benefits of treatment? What is the goal of treatment?
- Where will I have the chemotherapy and how long for? What access is required? Portacath? PICC line (see Chapter 7)?
- What side effects occur with this cancer treatment, short and long term? When do they occur? How long will they last? How do we manage them?
- Will I be able to work whilst on cancer treatment?
- What if I become unwell during chemo? And what do I look out for?
- What are my research trial options?
- What are the do's and don'ts through this treatment? Lifestyle? Alcohol? Exercise?
- Will this treatment affect my fertility or cause an early menopause?
- What if I don't want treatment?
- How am I monitored on treatment and how will I know that it is working?
- I'm not keen on the treatment offered after listening to and reading all the information, could I ask for a second opinion or are there other treatments available privately?
- How long will it take till I feel back to normal and recover?

Questions to ask your cancer nurse specialist

Many of the questions you would want to ask your surgeon or oncologist, you may find your specialist nurse is able to answer, and if they can't, they can ask and find out for you if you haven't got a meeting with your specialist doctor coming up. Other questions you may want to ask include:

- When is my next follow-up?
- What will surveillance entail, and will I have CEA monitoring, scans and colonoscopies?
- What do I do if I have any problems after treatment finishes?
- How can I reduce my risk of recurrence?
- How can I stay healthy during and after treatment?
- I'm worried about recurrence, what can I do?

Questions to ask your GP or family doctor

- What lifestyle changes should I be making to help with treatment?
- How can we manage my mental health?
- What will my recovery look like?
- How and when do I return to work – will I get a sick note?
- How can I cope with the side effects that treatment will bring?
- Where and how can I apply for benefits or financial support?

I've left a page below for you to write any questions you may have as they arise while reading, or while going through treatment and beyond.

6

Surgery, stomas and self-help – oh my!

Before we start, let's recap on the colon and rectum with a little anatomy lesson first, if we may.

Anatomy

Understanding the anatomy of the colon and rectum (Figure 6.1) helps us understand which operation may be performed, depending on the tumour's location. We talked about the functions of the colon and rectum in the previous chapter.

Types of endoscopic and surgical treatment for colorectal cancer

There are a number of ways to treat colorectal cancer. It all depends on where the cancer is, its size and whether or not it has spread.

Endoscopic mucosal resection (EMR) and endoscopic submucosal dissection (ESD)

If you have a very small, early-stage cancer, or a cancer that appears to arise within and is confined to an identifiable polyp, it may be possible for it to be removed via specialist endoscopy techniques – known as an endoscopic mucosal resection or an endoscopic submucosal dissection (ESD). This allows removal of abnormal tissue without the need for open surgery. The tissue will be sent to the pathologist to ensure the abnormal tissue has been removed in its entirety, and will help provide information about whether the procedure has been successful in treating the cancer.

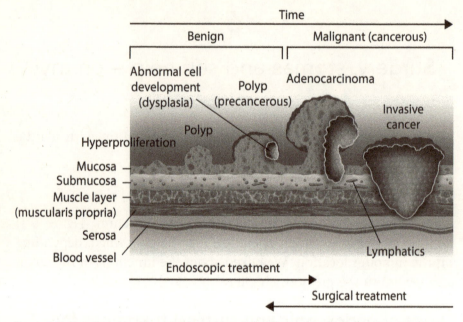

Figure 6.1   Development of a polyp (benign) and transformation to a cancer over time.

Only selected cases will be suitable to undergo an EMR or an ESD to treat cancer. The advantage of an endoscopic approach to treat early cancer is that the procedure is minimally invasive, carried out during a colonoscopy or sigmoidoscopy as mentioned earlier. It can be performed as an outpatient, the recovery time is significantly shorter, and there is significantly less pain during the recovery period when compared to conventional surgery. Disadvantages are that the tumour may not be completely removed, and there are risks of causing significant bleeding or perforation (an unwanted hole in the bowel) during the procedure.

In addition, anyone who undergoes EMR or ESD treatment for cancer will need to be very closely monitored, usually through a combination of scans and repeated endoscopies, to ensure the cancer does not recur.

Surgery for colon cancer

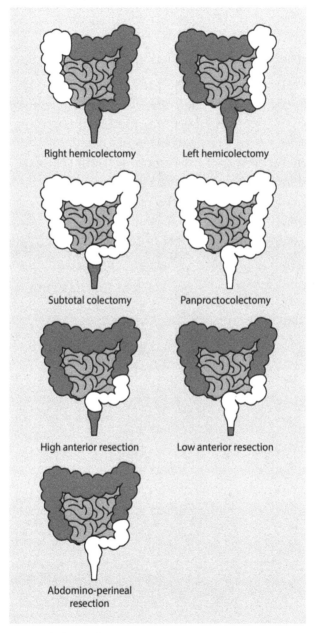

Right hemicolectomy

Left hemicolectomy

Subtotal colectomy

Panproctocolectomy

High anterior resection

Low anterior resection

Abdomino-perineal
resection

Figure 6.2 Types of surgery
Source: Bowel Cancer UK

If the tumour is too big or has invaded deeper than the layer of the submucosa (see Figure 6.1), then surgery will be recommended. The surgery offered will depend on where in the bowel your tumour is situated (see Figure 6.2). Here are the common types of surgery that can be performed:

- **Right hemicolectomy:** if the tumour is on the right side of the bowel, the right side of the colon, called the ascending colon, will be removed. If the tumour is in the middle of the colon, the surgeon will perform a right extended hemicolectomy.
- **Left hemicolectomy:** if the tumour is in the left side of the colon, the descending colon will be removed.
- **Subtotal colectomy:** removal of all of the colon.
- **Proctocolectomy:** removal of the colon and rectum.
- **Panproctocolectomy:** removal of the colon, rectum and anus.

These last three operations are usually offered if a patient has the genetic condition FAP or UC, or has tumours in multiple sites.

Anterior resection surgery for rectal cancer

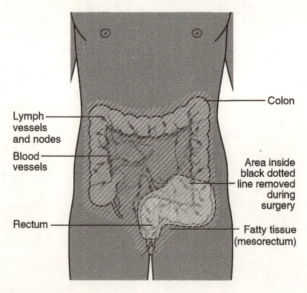

Figure 6.3 Anterior resection

This image was produced by Macmillan Cancer Support and is reused with permission. Additional labels have been used.

For rectal cancers or cancers in the sigmoid colon, you will be offered an anterior resection. Ironically, this was the first surgery I witnessed in a hospital theatre on my first day of placement at medical school, and it was also the operation I underwent. This operation aims to remove a segment of your bowel known as the sigmoid colon with part of your rectum, as well as the associated blood supply surrounding lymph glands. The remaining part of your rectum will be reconnected to your colon, or a temporary ileostomy will be performed. The procedure may be either a high anterior resection or low anterior resection as in Figure 6.4, depending on how much of the rectum is removed.

In 1982, Professor Richard J. Heald developed the technique that is now known as total mesorectal excision (TME). This not only removes the tumour, it also removes the surrounding fat and lymph nodes. This reduces the risk of local recurrence of the tumour to 3 per cent, compared with 20 per cent previously. As a result, everyone now with rectal cancers has a TME with their anterior resection.

I had a low anterior resection and TME, with a temporary ileostomy. Like many who have this operation, I'm left with a combination of symptoms called LARS (lower anterior resection syndrome) as a result of the procedure, and I'll talk more about this later in the book. Those who have a low anterior resection may also experience sexual dysfunction on top of this.

Colo-anal J pouch surgery

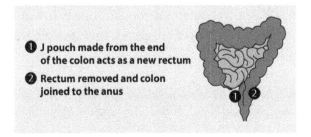

Figure 6.4   Colo-anal J pouch surgery
Source: Bowel Cancer UK

For cancers in the lower part of the rectum, the surgeon will remove most of the rectum, and subsequently join the end of the colon to the anus. This join is called a colo-anal anastomosis. Sometimes the surgeon uses the end of the colon to make a pouch, called a J pouch (colo-anal J pouch surgery, Figure 6.4). This will act as a storage facility (like the rectum previously) for stool, before you go to the toilet. A stoma may be required while the join between the anus and colon heals.

Abdomino-perineal resection (APeR of the rectum)

If the cancer is very low down in the rectum, your surgeon will need to remove the rectum and anus. This operation involves removing the whole of your rectum and anal canal. Your anus will be removed and the skin around the back passage will be closed, leaving a permanent stoma.

Pelvic exenteration

I'd like to introduce you to Nat who aged just 36 had a pelvic exenteration after her diagnosis of stage 4 CRC. By the time Nat was diagnosed, she was really quite ill, had lost a significant amount of weight, was suffering with constant back pain; her periods had stopped and her bowels had stopped working. Prior to her surgery she underwent a punishing course of chemo-radiotherapy, that successfully shrank her tumours so they could be operated on, followed by further chemo. Unfortunately the COVID pandemic hit and her surgery was delayed; she was given second line chemo-therapy as a holding measure until eventually she could have the treatment she needed, facilitated by a complex cancer clinic at St Mark's, a specialist bowel hospital in London. Nat went on to have the mother of all bowel cancer surgeries, and as you read her words below you will see why.

Nat @iamnatwoodward
My cancer was basically filling my pelvis and growing into my spine, pelvic bone, reproductive organs and lymph nodes. The tumours were inside and outside of my bowel and had grown back into my spine, forward into my vagina, and it was inoperable – they didn't think they would be able to cure me.

Three months after my initial gruelling chemo-radiotherapy, I had a scan that showed that my cancer had responded remarkably well, better than they had hoped, and had almost completely disappeared. It felt like a miracle!

I had further chemotherapy and another scan. Unfortunately, this one showed that the tumour had already started to grow back, and had started growing a little higher up the bowel too.

I was told that my complex and recurrent cancer needed to be treated by a specialist hospital, so I was referred to the Complex Cancer Clinic at St Mark's Hospital, the national bowel hospital. In February 2020, I was told that in order to stand a chance at having a future I would need an operation called pelvic exenteration.

All pelvic exenterations vary greatly, depending on the person, and the cancer and which organs are affected. My exenteration was very extensive, though I have met people who have had even more extensive ones than mine. My surgeons would need to remove my ovaries, fallopian tubes, uterus, cervix, vagina, rectum, anus, a section of my sacral spine and five spinal nerves, my left piriformis muscle, left pelvic side wall. By this time the cancer had spread to my left ureter (the tube that connects your kidney to your bladder) so they needed to cut the cancer out of my ureter and then re-implant the healthy part of my ureter back into my bladder, which of course meant cutting into my bladder. It would probably have been easier for them to remove my bladder, but my amazing surgeon knew how much I wanted to try to keep it, so that I would only have one stoma for life.

I didn't even know it was possible to live having had so much of you removed, it was so much to get my head around. I knew that I had missed my chance of conceiving a child naturally, but I had met cancer patients who had had an egg donor and had still carried and birthed their babies. I had naïvely been holding out hope for that. Finding out that they would need to remove my womb, my rectum and anus and I would have a stoma for the rest of my life, however long that may be, was really, really devastating. There was a strong chance I wouldn't have the use of my left foot due to the spinal surgery. There was the impact on my relationship, and on me as a young woman getting her sex organs cut out. A big part of me wondered if my life would be worth living afterwards, and if it would be worth surviving at all – but luckily the will to live kicked in pretty quickly and I agreed to the surgery. It was my only chance and I had to take it.

My surgery took 12 hours, with multiple surgeons working on me that day. For part of my surgery they had to lay me face down (prone), and the procedure was completed by a plastic surgeon who had to reconstruct the whole underneath of me, using most of my right buttock.

The recovery was brutal, and I was in hospital for a month.

Life after pelvic exenteration isn't easy, however for some of us it is our only chance at having more life and so, in my mind, the challenges I face daily, the things I grieve for, the things I have lost, the chronic pain I live with... none of it compares to the joy of having more life and making more memories with my loved ones.

I'm so happy to say that I'm now two years post-surgery and I am still getting scans that show no evidence of active disease. It is a place nobody thought I'd reach when I was first diagnosed.

I am forever indebted to my surgical team and family. I make sure I live each day to the full, despite the physical challenges I face, and I am so very grateful for every single day of life they have given me.

As Nat's story explains, pelvic exenteration is a radical surgical treatment that removes all organs from a person's pelvic cavity, potentially including the bladder, rectum, anus and urethra, as well as all the female reproductive organs (womb, cervix, ovaries and vagina). It is used to treat advanced colorectal cancer but can be used for the treatment of other cancers. There are different types of pelvic exenteration surgery and a surgeon may not know what type of pelvic exenteration is needed until they start the surgery. This is all dependent on the type of cancer the patient has, where the cancer is in the pelvis and if the patient has received any treatments in the past. The patient is likely to be left with a permanent stoma and potentially a urostomy (a bag collecting urine). The back passage will be sewn up.

How will the surgery be performed?

Depending on the operation, surgery can be performed in three different ways:

- **Open surgery:** one incision or cut is made from below your breast bone down your abdomen.
- **Laparoscopic surgery:** otherwise known as keyhole surgery. Three to four small incisions are made and a thin tube with a camera and light is passed through one incision, and instruments through the other, to perform the surgery. Generally, recovery is quicker, with a reduction in length of hospital stay, reduction in pain post-operatively and minimal scarring. It's important to understand that sometimes keyhole surgery needs to be converted to open surgery if technically difficult.
- **Robotic surgery:** this method is not currently available in all countries, but is increasingly being used. Like laparoscopic surgery, it is also minimally invasive and uses a camera. However, the surgeon will sit away from the patient, operating a robotic machine which has four arms, via a console. Stan shares his experience of robotic surgery in Chapter 21.

Decisions regarding which approach will be taken will be dependent on your surgeon and the hospital at which you are having your surgery, and questions can be directed to your hospital team regarding this.

Surgery for bowel obstruction or a 'blocked' bowel

Meet Lauren. She was diagnosed with bowel cancer aged 33. She shares the story of how her bowel cancer was eventually discovered – through a life-threatening blockage of her bowel.

Lauren, like Nat, did present multiple times with symptoms before a diagnosis was reached. Lauren's symptoms started with constipation, which then worsened when she was pregnant. Fatigue was a feature during the pregnancy, and unfortunately her symptoms were thought to be pregnancy related. She had several laxatives, including enemas with no real great effect, until things escalated and deteriorated.

Lauren (@house_of_fresa)

One night, I started vomiting and just couldn't stop. I couldn't leave the bathroom. I had also now stopped passing wind.

In the early hours of the morning, I called myself an ambulance as I knew something was seriously wrong with me. The ambulance came and the paramedic agreed that there was definitely something underlying that hadn't been explored. The gynaecology team were called and they checked baby's heartbeat, did a scan and then discharged me back to the surgical team. When I heard I might be discharged, I refused to leave the hospital. I knew there was something seriously wrong and I knew it needed to be investigated.

I was transferred to a side room off the gynaecology ward. I remember a nurse asking for a urine sample and it was such a dark colour, I had never seen anything like it, it was practically red! I hadn't managed to eat or drink anything for more than 24 hours, so I was immediately put on to a drip. Soon after, a colorectal surgeon came to see me and did a rectal exam (he later told me that he felt something then and there, and was deeply concerned).

I was sent for a colonoscopy and that's when it all got very serious. After seeing the colonoscopy, the surgeon immediately started to scrub up. He told me to ring my husband and tell him to come. As we were in the throes of the second lockdown, he would only be able to see me very briefly, and it was only because this was an emergency.

I needed stoma surgery ASAP. The surgeon said later that another 24–48 hours and my bowel would have completely ruptured, causing peritonitis and death. When I heard these words I felt so let down, angry with every medical professional I had come in to contact with over the last five months.

Hours later, in a room by myself, I was told that there was no heartbeat and that my baby had died. I was crushed. I had to phone my husband and tell him over the phone that our son had passed away. It was horrific.

After two more days in hospital, we were told that the blockage in my bowel was caused by a cancerous tumour in my rectum which had already spread to my liver. The surgeon explained that the next steps would be a course of radiotherapy along with oral chemotherapy, chemotherapy treatment and then hopefully surgery to remove the tumour and the mets on my liver.

If I could give any advice it would be: please listen to your body. Mine was crying out to let me know that something was wrong and unfortunately it took a long time for me to be heard. I wish I had been more forceful sooner. Please see your doctor as soon as you notice a change or symptoms which you are concerned about.

Lauren's story is devastating. I will highlight two particularly key aspects: firstly, that there are patients who present in pregnancy, and the symptoms experienced may be similar to those experienced in pregnancy. Secondly, some patients with advanced cancer may present with a 'blocked bowel' or bowel obstruction secondary to the tumour. This is a surgical emergency. Studies vary, but it is likely that 15–29 per cent of patients present acutely with bowel obstruction and this percentage is higher in the younger age groups, where patients are often diagnosed later, having presented later or been turned away, their symptoms being attributed to other causes.

Previous surgery or radiotherapy increases the risk of bowel obstruction too. When the bowel becomes partially or totally blocked, digested food can no longer pass freely through it, resulting in a patient experiencing the following symptoms.

Symptoms of bowel obstruction

- Severe, cramping tummy pain that comes and goes as your bowel tries to contract to move food through the blockage
- Feeling that food is getting stuck as it moves through the stomach
- Feeling sick
- Vomiting large amounts (undigested food and bile)
- Constipation, and not passing any wind
- Feeling bloated and full

Patients should seek medical attention promptly if they display any of these symptoms.

Once a bowel obstruction is confirmed (usually on a CT scan of the abdomen), the obstruction needs to be relieved as soon as possible.

Sometimes a colonoscopy is performed and an expandable hollow metal tube called a stent is passed through to bypass the blockage temporarily before surgery. Surgery is often required to remove the bowel with the blockage that contains the cancer, and a temporary or permanent stoma may be required.

I know what surgery I'm having – what next?

You know the surgery that may be on offer, you have your surgery date – or you are thinking of helping a loved one pack their hospital bag, or buying them some practical items to take into hospital.

What to take in your hospital bag

My initial packing included everything bar the kitchen sink. However, for the more sensible, the list may include:

- Phone or a tablet
- Books or magazines
- Headphones
- Phone charger with a long cable – my plug didn't quite reach.
- Small amount of cash
- Eye mask and ear plugs – essentials!
- Underwear – lots of it
- Glasses or contact lenses
- Medications you usually take
- Comfortable soft pyjamas, loose-fit jogging bottoms and sweat-shirts or night gowns
- Dressing gown and slippers
- Shaving equipment
- Pads in case of faecal leakage
- Wash bag, toothbrush, small towel, make-up if you wear it – when I started applying make-up, it was a sign I was getting better!
- No valuables.

Preparing for treatment emotionally and physically

So, it's on. A date for surgery, chemotherapy and/or radiotherapy has been written in the sand. It can be nerve wracking and you're probably thinking, 'How on earth do I prepare for this?'

None of us planned for a cancer diagnosis, but what we, and you, can do is to take some of the control back. This can have a positive impact on your emotional wellbeing, so it's an important step to take before treatment starts. It pays to get organized beforehand, as you will need to rest and recover when you are discharged home. If, however, you don't feel mentally or physically up to it, then if you are fortunate enough to have people around you to help, delegate away.

I automatically went into both military and nesting modes when it came to getting on with things. At the eleventh hour, I decided that my lounge needed redecorating (thank heavens for my husband and friend C humouring me and helping me achieve that). I busied myself with distractions, rallying the troops, giving instructions and talking openly to friends and family about what we might find useful, to help ease what was going to be a difficult process. I decided I needed a declutter and, most importantly, I needed to attend to one more challenge that had been planned for a while, before I was out of action for a period of time, and unable physically to achieve it. I'm so grateful for my hospital team, family and friends supporting this last challenge, climbing Mount Mulhacén in the Sierra Nevada just a week after diagnosis and a week before surgery, because I knew mentally I would have been crushed if I hadn't been able to do it, and that I'd start my treatment on the back foot. Doing whatever you need to do to enable you to feel you are in the driving seat is crucial as you go forwards into treatment.

Below are some tips about how you might need practical support or how you would practically support someone faced with cancer.

Top 10 tips to prepare for treatment

1 Prehabilitation (see Chapter 11). Take regular exercise to ensure you are in the best state of physical health possible prior to operation day, staying fit and active as part of prehabilitation. If you're a smoker, consider stopping as this will reduce your risk of complications after surgery. Ask your doctor to signpost you to sources of help.

2 Stock up your fridge or freezer and batch cook if you can or, if people offer help, suggest a food rota (something that I found priceless). Be sure to tell them of any allergies and dietary requirements – for example, if you will be having a stoma. Set up online shopping.

3 Organize childcare if there is any doubt you will be able to manage. I was out of action completely for the first week post-op, and for the first week of each chemo cycle. Let the school know, so the teachers can look out for any change in your child's behaviour and offer them extra emotional support. If you are a carer, find help to support the person you care for when you are unable to, this is not always easy to predict I know. Pet care – ask friends or family, local vets if they know of any volunteering schemes or charities. You may find yourself nesting. I certainly did – cleaning the house from top to bottom. Work out how you spread out the housework, or even pay a cleaner if you can afford it.

4 Talk to your employer if you need or want to discuss your diagnosis, let them know how long you might be out of action and tie up any loose ends admin wise.

5 Pack your hospital bag, whether for an in-patient stay or for day-case treatment.

6 Prepare for your physical appearance to change. Look for products that are safe to use during chemotherapy, for example skin care/hair care. Possibly order a wig if needed.

7 Take a look at your home set-up. Can you access the toilet easily? I invested in an electric blanket to help with the nerve pain induced by the cold. Can you make a nice clean environment for when you're in bed or in the lounge resting? Can you get snacks and water easily? Do you need a box for medications?

8 Invest in some key products that may help reduce side effects, like urea-based cream for capecitabine chemo, ski gloves, scarves and thick bed socks for oxaliplatin, and so on.

9 Financial issues: cancer can be expensive – even just thinking about paying for hospital parking, needing to buy things to make treat-ment easier, potentially working less or not working at all. You may be eligible for a variety of benefits – speaking to a cancer team like Macmillan who can help signpost you to what you need to do may be beneficial. You also may have taken out income protection or crit-ical illness insurance policies or have cover from work in the event of a serious medical illness such as cancer, and it's important to get in touch with them to see what you are potentially eligible for. Private pensions also may allow you to take money out early if you are diag-nosed with cancer. There is often free car parking when attending for treatment, so ask your ward what you may be entitled to.

10 If you live alone or think you may need extra support at home, please let your CNS know.

There is also the emotional side to consider. There has been no time to process the fact that you have cancer, let alone the treatment to come, and your emotional wellbeing may be fragile. Take the time to look after yourself prior to treatment, and let others be there for you, to lean into, so you can embark on treatment with as much positivity as you can, under these difficult circumstances.

Here are some top tips on getting emotionally ready for treatment.

Top 10 tips to prepare emotionally for treatment

1 Be clear about your plan. Hopefully you took someone with you to the appointment to discuss the plan but if you have any thoughts or questions that arise afterwards, do get in touch with your specialist cancer nurse who can help.
2 Stay active and as fit as you can.
3 Eat a healthy, balanced diet. No matter what treatment, what stage of cancer you have, these pillars are so important for your physical and mental health and your wellbeing, and can improve your quality of life. I'll talk more about this in Chapter 16.
4 Set up a support group through WhatsApp, email or social media of friends and family, to keep people updated in one place if that's what you choose – or where you can ask for help, a shoulder to cry on, and so on. Tap into this support guilt-free. Equally if you are allergic to flowers or your fridge is full, you can point out what you don't need. People want to help, and it's always easier if they are told what to do or not to do.
5 Treat yourself. New pyjamas, new lipstick, new slouchy pants, anything to make you feel comfortable – a little bit of self-care can go a long way.
6 Recognize what you may find relaxing and invest in self-care – music, apps such as Headspace or Calm, cooking, podcasts, box sets, meditation, mindfulness.
7 Plan for what you can; don't worry about what you can't.
8 Talk to someone who has been through it. But remember, everyone's experience of cancer is unique and what works for them may not work for you. However, talking can also help alleviate fear, concerns and anxieties about upcoming treatment as well as the uncertainty moving forwards. It helps you feel less alone. Reach out through the friend of a friend, through social media searches, to support groups or through charity pages.
9 Read affirmations – I had a beautiful handmade tree gifted to me full of affirmations written by all those around me. Some of those quotes I have gifted to you through this book, in the hope they will

lend themselves to someone else who needs them right now. 'You are stronger than you know, braver than you think and more loved than you can imagine.'

10 See your doctor if you are struggling and feel the emotional burden is so much that it's impacting your mental health. Seek treatment, and/or therapy or counselling. It's better to start early than wait for treatment to start, and for things to become even harder.

Pre-surgery

You will be invited to a pre-operative assessment where you will be asked lots of questions pertaining to your health, given an examination, further tests and an anaesthetic review if needed, depending on your pre-operative health status and your medical history.

You will be given instructions as to what to eat and drink prior to surgery and when to be nil by mouth. If you are not diabetic, you may be given a drink called a preload, a sugary drink. Benefits include reducing your risk of infection, aiding recovery, helping wounds heal and reducing sickness. You may also be asked to take bowel prep – which clears out your bowel prior to surgery (see Chapter 3 for tips on how to make bowel prep more palatable). Please follow to the T any instructions you are given.

Ensure your bag is packed, ready to go.

Surgery day

You will be well looked after, but take someone with you if you can. Leave plenty of time so you are not adding to the stress and know that you and your team have got this. I had a lot of nervous energy, my anticipation levels were high and while I was wheeled into the anaesthetic room, silent tears trickled down my face. Thankfully I had a fantastic anaesthetist, old school, but kind and caring – he promised me a spinal block to help with my sciatica, too, and the panic fell away as the general anaesthetic washed through my veins and I was ready to say farewell to cancer.

What can I expect after surgery?

Of course, everybody's experience after surgery is different, but it might help you to know how things went for me. Once the surgery was completed, I was returned from recovery to the ward and the following 20 hours were a blur. Nurses checking my stoma, my catheter, my pain relief, my pulse, my blood pressure – usually with murmurs and sighs over my blood pressure (I always have a low blood pressure), filling me with fluids through my veins. The constant beeping of machines. All in a drug-fuelled haze. Interestingly, I felt pangs of hunger and decided to opt for stoma-friendly macaroni cheese. Salivating at the thought, I could feel my belly gurgle. After eating, I waited with anticipation for a volcanic eruption, in my new designer bag ... but nothing really happened for a while. One of the milestones post-operatively is the bowel working again. Another is the removal of your catheter and being able to urinate. And gradually, as my bowel began to wake up, I began to panic a little as the bag filled up, with gas or with waste products, and I called for the nurses to help me, and settle my fears – while the stoma nurse came daily to see how I was managing, and to help with this significant transition.

I had been told that there was protocol for post-operative recovery, as part of the Enhanced Recovery Programme, designed to return you to full health as quickly as possible. Research shows that after the operation, it is better to begin eating food and drink fluids early on, to have the optimal pain relief on board, and get moving quickly. This has the added benefit of reducing the likelihood of complications post-operatively. However, for me the thought of getting out of bed was just too much the first day. For someone who is so active, and usually can't keep still, I thought the surgical team were frankly having a laugh (and was less than impressed as a patient at their evidence base). I felt so unwell, lightheaded and washed out and the pain on moving was significant. However, as a doctor, I knew we had to get on top of the pain to get me up and mobile, so with the help of the pain management team, my medications and side effects were reviewed, and I was determined to get going. And lo and behold, once the pain was controlled, I had consumed some calories and added in some broken sleep, my first trip to the toilet for a wee without a catheter was on day two. This honestly seemed like a marathon as I waddled precariously across the ward, my bottom hanging out. I didn't care, I was the youngest on the ward by far and had apparently bonded with the other women in the ward over our various bowel- and poo-related tales.

I found that after the operation there wasn't much time for languishing. The array of therapists and specialists, with visitors on top of that, and the lady screaming all night for 'Derek' next to me – well, it wasn't the most restful place to be. I sat and listened to the 'You, Me and the Big C' podcast, trying to make sense of what had just happened, opening my bloodshot eyes to the chaos of cancer, in between episodes of pressing my morphine pump in the hope of some pain relief.

With regard to the stoma, I felt terribly under-confident and nervous about its presence. I had been given stomas to practise with at home, before the surgery, but having one of your own was a whole different ball game. The panic about how I was going to manage this entity started mounting. The nurses on the ward were utterly wonderful (and overworked). They just didn't stop. My stoma started to have a mind of its own and the bag started inflating. I'm not sure the green smoothie I asked my brother to buy me the day before was such a good idea, but I was desperate for something other than beige food. It was apparent in my drug-fuelled haze, even as a doctor, I had no idea what I was doing.

There was also the 'day three dip'. I wasn't even aware this was a thing, but one of the research doctors that I had enrolled in a study with told me all about this phenomenon, as he pulled round the curtain, and found me sobbing into my sheets. It is not unusual to find people very tearful on day three post operatively, as the potential sleep deprivation in hospital, the pain, the emotional stress, loneliness and fatigue start to take hold. I knew then I had to get home.

Remarkably, I was discharged on day four post op and was never so pleased to see my own bed. We had chosen to send the children to my parents-in-law; my operation coincided with half term as I didn't want them seeing how I was in hospital. It also allowed G to visit freely after work. They did indeed come and pick me up from the hospital, and I could already sense a little of their fear, that Mummy had changed and didn't look so fresh and was obviously in pain. Recovery went from strength to strength as the days passed at home, and my emotions ebbed and flowed, although my struggles with the stoma at times were real (we will talk stomas shortly). On day ten post op, my surgeon, Prof Rockall, and CNS, Angie, were pleased to see me walk into the consulting room, pain-free.

During this consult, after discussing how I had been faring since my discharge, I also made a personal request to have my stoma reversed prior to chemotherapy. This is an unusual decision and most keep their stoma for gut-related side effects from chemo. My stoma had a fairly high output, and I felt that physically and emotionally I would be better placed to start chemo if there was an option of having this reversed first. After an informed discussion, we agreed that I could have the stoma reversed prior to chemotherapy and I would need a special X-ray called a gastrografin enema to ensure my bowel had healed at the new join that had been made.

We also now had the results from the tumour which had been removed. You will have heard me mention radiological staging of the cancer prior to surgery – this is when the stage of the cancer is determined by scans and biopsy results only (see Chapter 3). Once the tumour has been removed, a pathologist will look at the cancerous cells to determine the size and give a more accurate staging of your cancer. If the cancer has spread to the lymph nodes, or it is an aggressive tumour and there is a high risk of it spreading to other parts of your body, you will be offered chemotherapy. My cancer was actually downstaged from a stage 3C rectal cancer to a stage 3B cancer as fewer lymph nodes were involved, after they were analysed post-surgery, than seen on initial scans. This was good news. Pre-surgery, the cancer was thought to have spread to four lymph nodes on MRI scans, however on closer inspection, there was only actually one lymph node affected. The fewer nodes affected, the better my outlook or prognosis, even though I had a locally advanced cancer.

From here, I was to be sent to my oncologist, Dr Stewart, to discuss treatment with chemotherapy and what this new staging meant for me in the weeks, months and years to come.

Stomas

Here, I'd like to guide you through the world of stomas, with a little help from my friends. People often don't know what they are and if they are told they need one, some may be horrified, whereas others have no idea what it may entail.

What is a stoma?

The word 'stoma' comes from the Greek word meaning 'mouth' or 'opening'. A stoma is a section of bowel which protrudes out through an opening on the abdomen's (tummy's) skin surface. Poo is then collected in a bag or pouch attached to your skin, which can be emptied and changed. There are different types of stomas.

Your surgeon will discuss the need for a stoma, and whether it will be permanent or a reversible measure (to allow the bowel ends or the anastomosis to join and heal once the tumour has been removed).

Waking up to a stoma is not easy. But it is an essential mechanism which can be life saving.

Figure 6.5 is a diagram of an ileostomy and colostomy and the differences between them. The colon is responsible for absorbing water, which is why what is produced by an ileostomy has a bigger volume than that of a colostomy as there hasn't been the opportunity for the water to be reabsorbed.

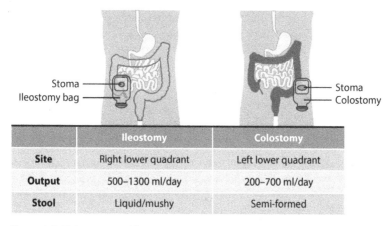

	Ileostomy	Colostomy
Site	Right lower quadrant	Left lower quadrant
Output	500–1300 ml/day	200–700 ml/day
Stool	Liquid/mushy	Semi-formed

Figure 6.5 Colostomy and ileostomy

Ileostomy

Over half of patients with a rectal tumour will have a temporary ileostomy or a 'defunctioning' ileostomy once their rectal tumour is removed. This allows time for the bowel to heal and reduces the risk of stool leaking out the bowel which would make you quite unwell. The amount of time patients may keep their stoma varies and can be anything from 3–12 months or longer, till they finish their treatment.

Depending on their surgery, others may require a permanent stoma. Below, Neil shares his experience of a permanent ileostomy formation. Neil had a history of Crohn's disease and was diagnosed with stage 2 bowel cancer at the age of 40. He underwent an open panproctocolectomy, removal of the anus and ileostomy formation at the same time.

Neil (@bigwoofa)

Cancer – I had about a month to process what was coming, which was hard. Will I die, has it spread, what treatment? Chemo? Then you are going to have a permanent ileostomy? What does that mean? A lot to process. I was married with a daughter about to leave primary school.

In the meantime I met the specialist stoma nurse and surgeon who talked me through what the op would be like and explained the jargon. At that point I was pragmatic, 'it's not happening just yet, so postpone any nerves until it's here'. Adrenaline kicked in.

On the day of admittance I became a wee bit anxious. The mood was light-hearted when I was brought a stoma pouch to try, filled with water. I didn't take the adhesive cover off and got soaked! The hours after my wife left were hardest. Will I wake up after the op? Shaving nipple to groin, I sobbed in the shower. The bowel prep had worked its magic and I was woken at 4 am for an enema – 'You would pay a lot for this!' the nurses joked.

The actual operation went well. Afterwards I had 48 hours of morphine-induced hallucinations and madness, then learnt that three things you don't want to do post operatively are: 1 cough; 2 be told anything funny; and 3 move. Of course all three happen and it was absolute agony. You control the pump, and it was a dose every five minutes with one click. I clicked it 100 times in five minutes!

It's crucial to get moving as soon as the nurses and surgeon say you can and I won't lie, you will hurt like you cannot believe and even sitting up is exhausting. But gradually each day you move a little more and the pain does recede.

A key thing your surgeon wants to see is that your new stoma is working, which can take several days if (as in my case) you have only the small intestine left. Post-operatively, the bowel enters a state of shock when it has been handled, and it takes some days to begin to work.

Once I was able to move a little easier, and various catheters and tubes into my stomach had been removed, I was told I couldn't leave until I could manage my own stoma. I was keen to do this, so my stoma nurse used the EDIP principle – explain, demonstrate, imitate (do it with the stoma nurse supervising) practise and the same again the next day until they were happy I could manage on my own. I got caught getting a nurse to help once and was told off!!

You will be given enough kit to last a week or so when you leave hospital, and information on stoma supply companies. What are they? Well, there are many manufacturers of ostomy products and you don't get these from the pharmacy, as specialist companies will receive your prescription and deliver them to your home, usually monthly. Most of these companies supply accessories that you will also need, like disposal bags, skin wipes, and other useful things to help you feel comfortable and keep your peristomal skin (the skin around your stoma) in good order – excoriated skin is very sore. You can choose the delivery company yourself or take a recommendation from your stoma nurse. I later changed mine, but not at first till I was more comfortable with everything and knew more about what I needed. It's worth noting that these companies often have in-house nurses to advise on issues.

Throughout this time and in the future, you will have access to your hospital stoma nursing team. I'm friends with mine 20 years on.

These days, I'm a BC advocate, speaker, and run corporate training for Macmillan on cancer in the workplace. Outside I swim in the ocean, rock climb, run and am in my local mountain rescue team. I do all I did before and more. That didn't happen straightaway, but it did gradually. Life has been good to me.

Once healed you can travel, airplanes are fine, you can even parachute if you want to! There is so much support. As someone once said, 'Don't die wondering' – just do it.

Holistic care is important, not just for the stoma and cancer but for the mind, too.

I've collected below some helpful tips from people like Neil and Andrea, who you heard from earlier in the book, for managing a stoma.

Tips: Managing with a stoma

- Take things one day at a time: be gentle with yourself – look in the mirror at your tummy, repeat a positive mantra about your body each day. It may help you to accept your new body as you try to focus on body positivity and how much your body has seen you through. Living with a stoma is about your mindset, and there will be good days and bad days and everything in between. The early days are the hardest but it does get easier. You don't have to love it, but you can learn to live with it.

- The 'fit': stoma bags are like shoes/clothes – you don't have to stick with the one brand or product you are assigned at the beginning. If it is not working for you, or it doesn't feel right, try other brands: different sizes, different colours – it's all personal preference. Your stoma nurse can give you samples to try, and in the UK, your family doctor can continue to prescribe them.
- Self-praise: give yourself a little cheer after changing the bag on your own in the first months. It's a big achievement. You'll be changing it within five minutes and with your eyes closed in no time. I know I struggled initially and my husband and daughter even used to help!
- Rehabilitation and exercise: this is crucial after surgery and stoma formation. Take baby steps at first – do only what the hospital physio or stoma nurse advise you to. Once home keep up the routine they suggest, ask questions if unsure. It will be several weeks before you can drive (if you do), and they will advise on what not to do as well. Unfortunately, the majority of patients undergoing stoma formation for colorectal cancer become less active, compared to before surgery, yet there are so many important reasons to exercise. The main concern is trying to avoid developing a parastomal hernia, a common complication (where another loop of bowel can push through the abdominal wall next to the hernia), and this is where participating in the right exercises is key. There are a number of ways to reduce the risk: restoring your core muscle strength first and foremost, strengthening your pelvic floor and back is absolutely pivotal, as well as learning how to lift correctly. Sarah Russell's *Bowel Cancer Recovery Toolkit* is a great read (details in the Useful Resources section) and will help you get back to fitness. She has a stoma herself and is a personal trainer.
- Support: when you leave hospital, be aware your mood can take a dive. Eat well, exercise, sleep and talk to people about how you are feeling. Neil would specifically suggest joining the IA (Ileostomy Association) if you have an ileostomy, or Colostomy UK if you have a colostomy. It's not expensive but they are experts in your new plumbing and have lots of help and advice, plus you'll hear about new product developments and there will be useful information on common problems. In addition, there is an online forum and telephone support for everything from sore skin, to sex, and anything else you can imagine.
- Diet: the dietician will give you lots of advice and tips; you need a balanced diet, ask them for help. Some individuals can eat most of what they did before, including fibre, although you should avoid vegetables that are not well cooked.

- **Leaks:** these do happen – more often in the first six months. They will lessen once your stoma size has settled (it often changes size, and shrinks down a little until your bowel has fully healed and recovered). Have some pre-cut stoma bags at the ready in case of a leak in the night as trying to cut a bag sleepily isn't fun! If you are persistently experiencing leaks, please let your stoma nurse know so they can try to help find a solution. Have a stoma changing bag with you always when you're out if the need arises. This should contain all the equipment needed to change your stoma: fresh underwear, wipes, bags, and the adhesive remover spray.
- **Dehydration:** it can be common to suffer with dehydration if you have an ileostomy. Symptoms include feeling tired, groggy and light-headed. It's important to mix up the drinks you consume and not just drink water. For example, milk, tea, coffee, squash, juice. On top of this, include a daily electrolyte drink (like Dioralyte) or add a pinch of salt into squash, which replaces salts and minerals lost through the stoma.
- **'Pancaking':** a term that I discovered early on with my stoma. It's where a vacuum occurs in the stoma bag, preventing the contents from dropping to the bottom of the bag so it all collects around the stoma site, a 'pancake'. Top tips include: inflating the bag beforehand by blowing a little air in, covering the filter with toilet paper, wearing loose fitting trousers/pants, greasing the inside of the bag with baby oil or olive oil, increasing fluid intake, or trying a different bag.
- **Support garments:** this is something I chose to wear after surgery for comfort. This can be in the form of supportive pants or a wide stoma belt which can make having a stoma more comfortable in the early days where my abdominal muscles needed support after surgery.
- **Calamine lotion:** this does wonders for your skin – if your skin is sore from leaks or just sore from your bag, pop some calamine lotion on, wait for it to dry and you can still pop a bag on.
- **Hairdryer:** you can use a hairdryer on your bag after a shower or bath – set it to medium heat and it works a treat. Also give your bag a quick blast of the hairdryer when putting on a new one – the warmer the bag is, the better it will stick.
- **Sex:** if you are in or about to embark on a relationship, intimacy can cause some anxiety. Having sex is important and once a person has healed there is usually nothing to stop someone enjoying sex again. If there are problems, speak with your surgeon and stoma nurse. There can be surgical complications but they can usually be overcome (see Chapter 14). Then you can do all you did before and maybe more! But ideally with your ileostomy bag drained beforehand ... Neil points out: 'Occasionally accidents do happen, my

wife has occasionally knocked my pouch and it's come off, which can involve a shower and a change of sheet! Along with some giggling. My partner accepted me with my stoma. Where a stoma is cited as ending a relationship, then probably there were other issues beforehand.'

- Stoma nurse: if you are worried about something, ring and ask your stoma nurse. You should be able to work, exercise, have sex, swim, travel, eat a varied diet and thrive with a stoma. It shouldn't limit your life, and there are always other options if things aren't working out for you. Mine was a fount of knowledge and an absolute lifeline.

The way you feel and your outlook regarding the stoma will differ depending on whether your stoma is temporary or permanent. This is Nat, who we heard from earlier:

I had to have a stoma (colostomy) almost immediately, I didn't have much time to think about what this meant. I don't actually think I really knew what a stoma was so it was quite a shock when I woke up to see part of my intestine sticking out of my abdomen and attached to the outside. I felt quite positive about it all, mainly because I assumed the stoma would be temporary and would just help me get through my treatment to try to get on top of the cancer. I think it's quite different psychologically knowing that your stoma is temporary, playing its role through treatment, as opposed to when you are told that it will be with you for the rest of your life, which actually is my current reality. At that time, I just saw it as one step closer to getting better.

There is no doubt that stomas can be a handful and a huge life adjustment for anyone undergoing one. Ask for support if you are struggling – help is out there, so please don't feel alone.

7

Treatment options – 'What cocktail next?'

'It always seems impossible till it's done.'

Nelson Mandela

There are a number of other therapies that may be offered when it comes to the management of bowel cancer, aside from surgery. These include chemotherapy, radiotherapy, immunotherapy and targeted therapy – either as single agents or in combination. What people may not appreciate is that treatment can be given at different phases and the aim of treatment may vary according to the stage:

- **Curative treatment:** to remove the tumour completely, with the intent to be cancer-free.
- **Neoadjuvant therapy:** this is treatment given BEFORE the main treatment (surgery or radiotherapy) to help reduce the tumour bulk by shrinking it in size, and making it easier to remove surgically (e.g. chemo-radiotherapy for rectal cancer).
- **Adjuvant therapy:** treatment given AFTER surgery to mop up any cancer cells that may have escaped from the tumour, reducing the chance of recurrence.
- **Disease controlling or palliative treatment:** for metastatic CRC to try to control the disease for as long as possible and to relieve or lessen symptoms, but not to cure your cancer. This treatment aims to prolong and improve quality of life and to help you remain active for as long as possible.

When I was diagnosed with rectal cancer, there was a degree of uncertainty as to whether I would require chemo-radiotherapy before surgery or not, due to the position and size of my tumour. The majority of patients with my stage of cancer indeed do receive it.

After the multidisciplinary team meeting to discuss my case, I was involved in a discussion with my surgeon and oncologist who felt the case was borderline as to whether I would need chemo-radiotherapy first. On balance and in view of my age (and the potential for lifelong side effects, particularly from the radiotherapy), a collaborative decision was taken to take me to theatre for an examination under anaesthetic to see if the surgeon could remove the tumour entirely there and then without the need for any treatment beforehand. If he could, he would proceed with the operation, and if he wasn't confident, I would simply be closed up and sent for chemo-radiotherapy before any further surgery would be considered; a gamble, on balance, the team and I were willing to take.

What is chemo-radiotherapy?

Chemo-radiotherapy, a combination of both chemotherapy and radiotherapy. This treatment is usually given before surgery (neo-adjuvant chemo-radiotherapy) for rectal cancer. This can shrink the size of the tumour or lymph nodes and make it easier to remove surgically, as well as reducing the chance of the cancer returning locally at the same site. Rarely, chemo-radiotherapy is given after surgery (adjuvant chemo-radiotherapy), the hope is that it will destroy any remaining cancer cells if there is evidence from the tissue removed at surgery that some cancer cells may have been unexpectedly left behind.

Some patients may have this treatment as their main treatment, for example those with early small cancers or those unfit for surgery. Occasionally some cancers have completely responded to chemo-radiotherapy, and these individuals can then be enrolled in surveillance programmes without undergoing any surgery, which is incredible.

What are the main side effects associated with treatment?

All treatments may cause some side effects and as we go through all the modalities of treatment I'll describe some of them to you, from both my own experience and the experience of others. You may find these descriptions helpful and together with the help of Dr Stewart, my oncologist, and Angie, my CNS, we have some helpful hints to help you manage them at home. Nevertheless, in all cases it is essential if you do experience side effects that you let your specialist nurse or doctor know.

Capecitabine

This chemotherapy can be taken as part of chemo-radiotherapy before surgery, alone or after surgery in combination with other agents. It comes in the form of a characteristic pink tablet, taken twice a day. Once seen, never forgotten. The dose and number of pink tablets consumed is weight dependent.

DPD (dihydropyrimidine dehydrogenase) testing: before capecitabine is started, a blood test will be carried out to check for something called 'DPD deficiency'. This occurs in about 3–5 per cent of people – it means that the drug is broken down more slowly so lower doses are required to prevent serious side effects.

The general side effects of chemotherapy and their management are discussed below. There are also some side effects that are specific to this drug, but may vary between individuals.

Hand–foot syndrome (palmar–plantar erythrodysesthesia syndrome or PPE)

More than 50 per cent of patients taking this chemotherapy will experience this side effect. I certainly did when I took it in combination with another chemotherapy agent which I'll discuss later. Small amounts of this medication leak out of the blood vessels into the surrounding tissues, causing damage.

Soreness, redness and peeling of the skin on the palms and feet, which can cause pain, pins and needles, tingling, burning, itching and dryness, are common symptoms of this condition.

In severe cases, skin can peel off, blisters, sores or ulcers may form, and it may be difficult to walk or use your hands.

Tips: Managing hand–foot syndrome (PPE)

- Avoid hot showers and baths (reducing the leakage of medication into the tissues around them).
- Use skin products that contain 10 per cent urea three times a day as well as after handwashing to protect the skin. Studies show that this decreases the incidence of hand–foot syndrome for the first six weeks of treatment. I used Udderly Smooth. Applying regularly throughout the day is key. Other products recommended were Nursem and Eucerin products, both containing urea as the active ingredient.

- Keep pressure off the hands and feet. Avoid massaging or rubbing the feet or hands. Avoid using knives or DIY tools with repetitive movements.
- Apply ice packs – this is difficult if you are using this chemotherapy with another agent called oxaliplatin, where you cannot touch anything cold due to nerve pains – more on this later.
- Keep legs and feet elevated when resting.
- Wear slippers or soft socks.
- Pat, rather than rub, your feet dry.
- Avoid harsh chemicals from detergents on the skin.
- If your symptoms are severe, please talk to your specialist and they may consider lowering the dose.
- Pyridoxine – vitamin B6 supplementation – we don't know for sure if this helps with the neuropathy, but it won't do any harm if used.

Other more non-specific symptoms include:

Tiredness

During your chemo-radiotherapy treatment you may find that you feel very tired. Listen to your body, and if necessary, allow yourself extra time to rest.

Diarrhoea

I certainly remember the loose bowels when taking capecitabine. There was one particular occasion I thought I had a stomach bug and ended up needing the toilet at least 15 times. Remember, this is severe if you need the toilet more than four to six times in 24 hours. The advice is to stop taking your capecitabine tablets and telephone the Triage Service, sometimes known as the 'oncology treatment hotline', for advice immediately. Each hospital will have this service and it's important to have these details stored safely somewhere in case you need advice or help. We will look at ways to manage diarrhoea symptoms later in this chapter.

Constipation

If you are receiving capecitabine and the tumour has yet to be removed, you may get constipation and sometimes overflow diarrhoea as a result. Some people, rarely, may experience bowel obstruction.

Feeling sick (nausea)

Try to eat within 30 minutes of taking the capecitabine. I suffered heartburn taking these tablets, which contributed to my nausea. Eat little, but often.

Loss of appetite

Sickness, tiredness and taste changes contribute to a loss of appetite.

Mouth ulcers (stomatitis)

If you get any pain, redness, swelling or sores in or around your mouth you should let your medical team know. Looking after your oral hygiene, drinking plain fluids, avoiding citrus foods such as lemons and oranges, and chewing gum can help the mouth stay moist. Difflam mouth spray can be helpful too.

Changes in your blood

Your chemotherapy can sometimes affect your bone marrow, which produces different types of blood cells. If the number of blood cells in your body gets too low you may feel more tired and run down. You may also be more likely to get an infection or have a high temperature (fever). Because of this, regular blood tests will be arranged for you.

Effects on the heart

Rarely it can cause cardiac issues or side effects to the heart and its function. Please see section below.

It is important you contact your specialist or your hospital's oncology treatment hotline if you have any queries, but it is particularly important if you are experiencing any of the following on any type of chemotherapy:

- Suddenly feeling unwell
- A temperature greater than 37.5°C
- Any unexplained bruising or bleeding
- Diarrhoea for more than 24 hours
- Unrelieved shortness of breath
- Mouth ulcers that stop you eating or drinking

There are many other small print and rarer side effects, and these will all be given to you prior to starting treatment. I found the information given to me from my oncology team and the leaflets regarding each drug I took from the Cancer Research UK website the most helpful at the time and I avoided Dr Google to prevent any excess anxiety regarding treatment.

Radiotherapy

Radiotherapy is a method of treatment that uses carefully calculated and measured doses of radiation. Pelvic radiotherapy destroys cancer cells in the area where it is given, and is a potential treatment option for rectal cancer. It can also damage some normal cells, which in turn may cause side effects. When radiotherapy is given to the pelvic area, there are a lot of important surrounding structures that can also, unfortunately, be affected, causing a variety of side effects. If you are transgender and have had gender reassigning surgery, please check with your specialist if you're unsure what to look out for.

Radiotherapy can be given as part of treatment with surgery or chemotherapy or both. If your cancer is not curable, you may be given palliative radiotherapy to ease your symptoms.

Radiotherapy treatment is painless and only takes a few minutes, usually five days a week, for five weeks, or a short course alone for five days for one week.

For those taking it as part of chemoradiotherapy, you will be given radiotherapy five days a week, and on those days, you will be taking the capecitabine as well.

How is radiotherapy given?

Radiotherapy can be administered in the following ways.

External radiotherapy

If you receive external beam radiotherapy, this is delivered from a machine outside the body.

Internal radiotherapy (brachytherapy)

Internal radiotherapy means giving radiotherapy to the cancer from inside the back passage (rectum). The treatment gives a high dose of radiation to the cancer but very little to surrounding tissues. It can shrink the rectal cancer, relieve symptoms and help you feel more comfortable. It might slow the growth of the cancer and it can reduce pain.

There are two types of internal radiotherapy for rectal cancer:

- High dose rate brachytherapy (HDR)
- Contact x-ray brachytherapy (Papillion).

You might have contact x-ray brachytherapy:

- if you have an early cancer
- if your cancer measures less than 3 cm
- if you can't or don't want to have surgery.

This treatment is only available in a few hospitals.

What side effects can I expect from radiotherapy?

Meet Gemma. She was diagnosed with stage 4 cancer, aged 45, in August 2016. She underwent 12 cycles of FOLFOX chemo, followed by external beam radiotherapy with accompanying capecitabine prior to her bowel and liver resection for her tumours, and shares her experiences below.

Gemma (@gemmacollier5333)

Radiotherapy was actually the easiest part at the start. I drove myself in my new car (as I was given such a poor prognosis, I had a critical illness life insurance so bought myself my dream sports car. Note: do not spend any insurance payout too quickly – you may, as I did, 'survive' and regret such flippant purchases!) and managed to get myself to and from the hospital every day for five weeks.

The effects of radiotherapy are very much cumulative. If, like me, you have a number of weeks' treatment, be prepared to feel more and more tired as the treatment progresses. Another tip is to make enough time to park! Parking at hospitals is notoriously difficult at the best of times and it can reduce the stress levels if you leave good time to find a space.

Be prepared for the machine to break down and for treatment to be cancelled. Don't worry, a brief gap in treatment does not massively affect the outcome and the ones missed will be tagged on to the end. Take this into account if you are planning anything for when treatment finishes.

I also found reflexology very helpful during radiotherapy. Luckily, I had a friend who practised who came to the house but most cancer departments have treatment centres where volunteers will offer treatments. Use them!

I didn't suffer from sickness at all but there was, weeks in, a fine balance with some diarrhoea and then with taking medication for that swinging to constipation. My advice is, if it's not too bad, don't take medication as it can take you the other way which is painful!

During treatment you should see a nurse who will supply a vaginal dilator for use when you have pelvic radiotherapy. Use it! It will be painful and you may not feel that you want to do it, but it is necessary.

In general, apart from the tiredness, I coped pretty well so I booked a holiday for the week after treatment finished. Having a break is a good thing but be aware that the real after-effects only started about a week or so after I finished. I had tremendous pain, and symptoms not unlike the symptoms I had when first diagnosed: urgency to go, then not being able to, straining, and blood. I spent a lot of time weeping in the hotel bathroom. It was scary and had I known that this was normal then it would have helped. Don't take any codeine-related pain-killers – I was not aware that these can block you up, causing constipation, which in turn caused more pain, so use other types of pain relief. It does get better but it would have been less frightening had I been aware of the worsening of the symptoms after treatment had stopped.

Be aware that it is highly likely that radiotherapy to the pelvis will throw you into a medically-induced menopause. It was not highlighted enough to me, and I suffered a great deal, not knowing I was going through the menopause. Once I was put on HRT it was like magic.

Side effects from radiotherapy, as Gemma suggests, do not always occur straight away. They may develop during the course of treatment or in the days or weeks after treatment finishes. After you finish radiotherapy, the effects can worsen before they get better.

Meet Faith. She was diagnosed with stage 4 rectal cancer (T3N0M1– spread to the lungs) at age 47 and she gives an account of the side effects she experienced:

Faith (@faithwindsor)
Side effects didn't occur immediately but did include:

- Extreme fatigue
- Difficulty walking
- A very, very sore bottom
- Long-term pain in hips and back

I found the whole actual process relatively easy other than having to keep a full bladder!

Faith's tips include:

- Use very soft moist wipes for the loo from day one.
- Cooling gel. The bottom soreness lasted at least a month after treatment.

- Relax and rest as much as you possibly can. (Faith thinks she didn't rest enough and wished she had more from day one as she feels she suffers with long-term fatigue now.)

As Faith and Gemma suggested, side effects can include:

- **Tiredness and weakness:** tiredness after radiotherapy might carry on for some months and we will talk about fatigue later in the book.
- **Bowel dysfunction:** diarrhoea is the most common side effect. It usually starts during radiotherapy or after two weeks of treatment. Changes in bowel function occur due to damage to the bowel lining (which may cause bleeding), scarring of the large bowel making the bowel narrower and less flexible, as well as reducing its volume. This results in loose stool and the need to go urgently. Radiotherapy also affects the muscles that help store poo in the rectum which can cause incontinence. If radiotherapy affects parts of the small bowel, you may have diarrhoea or develop food intolerances.

Tips: Managing a change in bowel function during and after radiotherapy

- Keep a supply of loperamide (Imodium) in stock for diarrhoea.
- Fybogel or Normacol may help to bulk up the stools. Talk to your doctor before taking this.
- A study called the FIBRE study showed that a low-irritant, high-fibre diet can help. This diet can help reduce irritation to your bowel resulting in diarrhoea, bloating and wind caused by the pelvic radiotherapy. This involves cutting out insoluble fibres, but still eating plenty of food with soluble fibres which are digested more easily (see Chapter 2 for more on fibre types). It is a temporary measure through radiotherapy and it is important to still eat a wide array of foods, and when treatment ends, to reintroduce foods slowly. See Useful Resources for more information. Dieticians and specialist nurses can also help you manage this.
- Keep a food diary of which foods give you what symptoms.
- Try to drink at least 2–3 litres (3½ to 5½ pints) of fluids each day.
- For the sore bottom, use aloe vera, E45 or medihoney. Sudocrem can make it worse as it contains metal – so avoid!

- If you have any soiling or incontinence, tell your radiotherapy team. They will give you advice about coping with incontinence and looking after your skin.
- Avoid foods and drinks that give you wind, such as pickles, beans, curry and fizzy drinks.
- Do gentle exercise to help with wind. Or try taking charcoal tablets, which you can buy at the chemist; or drinking peppermint tea. These can affect other medicines, so always ask your doctor or pharmacist first.
- Please do speak to your cancer specialist nurse if you are passing blood from your bottom, waking up from your sleep to go to the toilet, suffering with urgency and rushing to the toilet, or have incontinence.

Further helpful hints can be found on the Macmillan website (see Useful Resources).

Other possible side effects from radiotherapy
Inflammation
This can cause anal irritation or pain in the back passage or during bowel movements (otherwise known as *radiation proctitis*). You may be asked to change your diet to control symptoms. You may also notice some discharge or bleeding from the back passage. Let your nurse or radiographer know if you have any of these problems.

Bladder dysfunction
Bladder changes can occur, such as pain when passing urine, as radiotherapy may cause damage to the tissue and blood vessels lining the bladder. You may need to urinate more often, and more urgently, just like a urine infection. This is called *radiation cystitis*. You may feel that you haven't emptied your bladder properly and need to go again as soon as you have just been. There may also be blood in your urine as the blood vessels are weaker and bleed more easily; please let your doctor know if this happens. Drinking plenty of fluids (2 litres a day), avoiding alcohol, fizzy and caffeinated drinks such as tea and coffee can help. A Radar key which gives you priority access to thousands of toilets in the UK would be useful. I received mine from my cancer specialist nurse. Alternatively, a 'Just can't wait' card is useful to obtain from Disability Rights UK or from Macmillan. If symptoms

persist, you may need a referral to an incontinence nurse, urologist or physiotherapist.

Redness and soreness of skin

Some people may experience a skin reaction, similar to sunburn around the bottom, while they are receiving radiotherapy. You may find that the skin in the treatment area becomes red, sore and itchy. Let your radiographer know if you have any redness or pain in the area being treated. They will be able to advise you on how to look after the skin in that particular area. Unperfumed moisturizing creams can be helpful. It is important to avoid exposing this area of skin to the sun's rays as this can increase the skin reaction.

Are there any long-term side effects?

There is also a small risk of long-term side effects – those lasting greater than three months. Side effects can sometimes also start months or years after radiotherapy. These are called *late effects*. Some of the symptoms above may also continue as long-term side effects including diarrhoea, radiation proctitis and bladder issues.

Meet Lauren. She talks about her experience of how she was given help to manage a potential long-term side effect that rarely is spoken about, with the help of a little purple box.

Lauren – 'My experience with radiotherapy and the little purple box'
About four weeks into starting radiotherapy, I noticed an appointment for 'feminine care' had been made for me. I didn't really think anything of it as I was led into a small room by a nurse. On the table next to her was a purple plastic box the size of a glasses case, and I was somewhat puzzled. The nurse proceeded to ask me how I was getting on with the side effects of treatment. I explained that other than feeling quite fatigued, I hadn't really had any other side effects and felt quite lucky.

She then sighed and replied, 'Well now I need to talk to you about more long-term side effects that will need addressing' and opened up the little purple box. I was in no way prepared for what she was about to say or just how much it would impact me even to this day.

She explained that when receiving radiation treatment to the pelvic area, muscles in the vagina can tighten somewhat even up to two years after and that at-home, self vaginal dilation is needed to keep the muscles stretched.

The reason it is important to do is the effects of radiation on your vaginal muscles can make it difficult to have sex comfortably after treatment and may also make it difficult for any future medical examinations.

Inside the purple box were four pink phallic-shaped lengths of plastic of vary-ing sizes which fit inside each other like a Russian doll. The nurse explained that I would need to use these each night for about 5/10 minutes. I was to start with the smallest size and graduate to the next size up as I saw fit. She also told me that if my husband and I were to have sex at any point, that would 'count as that day's dilation session'. A routine began and I started dilating as recommended.

In June 2022, I had extensive surgery to remove all the cancer in my body. I had a liver resection, full hysterectomy and the tumour removed from my rectum. Obviously during this time and the lengthy recovery period that fol-lowed, I neglected the little purple box and my husband and I were not having sex. When the time came to 'get back on the horse' as it were, we found that the muscles had completely tightened and sex was nigh on impossible! The purpose of the little purple box is so, so important, and I have written this to share my experience with others and to also shine a light on this issue. It is still very much part of my daily routine and it really is vital that I do it regularly. It is a side effect of radiotherapy which is still having an impact on my husband and I 18 months on.

Lauren has shared her experience of a debilitating symptom and its management in a very honest way. Below are some of the long-term side effects you could experience:

- **Sexual dysfunction:** pelvic radiotherapy can reduce libido in both men and women and there may be a change in sexual sensation. Men can experience a difficulty in getting an erection or problems with ejaculation following radiotherapy. It can also cause narrow-ing of the anal canal in both men and women.

- Women may develop vaginal dryness and shrinkage of the vagina. The skin inside the vagina can become thin and easily torn, caus-ing bleeding, discomfort and even sores inside the vagina, making sex painful. Radiotherapy for low rectal cancer can also cause the vagina to narrow. A member of the radiotherapy team will provide you with information on this and, if necessary, provide you with a device called a vaginal dilator to help manage this (which Lauren discusses above). You can start using these 2–8 weeks after treat-ment has ended to help prevent narrowing of the vagina. Gemma wants to also reiterate this message regarding the dilators:

Use them! It may be painful and you may not feel that you want to do it but it is necessary. I tried to keep up with the regime but I lapsed and unfortunately I had to have further surgery to try to 'open it up' again. Unfortunately, that did not work and it has greatly affected my ability to have sex (and enjoy it) without tremendous pain. Five years on and I still suffer.

Dr Stewart also mentions that vibrators can be used to help this as well as some evidence that clitoral stimulation may help too. It really is important to speak out about these symptoms, which are often not talked about, to get you the help that you need.

- **Early menopause:** pelvic radiation causes menopause by stopping the ovaries from working and producing oestrogen. The symptoms and risks are the same as those of a natural menopause and I will talk later in much greater depth about this important side effect and complication, as well as its management, as no one should have to suffer in silence! Pre-menopausal women receiving pelvic radiotherapy may want to explore any fertility preservation options (before starting treatment).
- **Other cancers:** all radiation treatments very slightly increase the risk of other cancers.
- **Weaker pelvic bones or tiny fractures in the bones:** also known as pelvic insufficiency fractures. This condition increases the chance of small cracks and fractures developing due to a change in density of the bones in the area that has received radiotherapy. Menopause in women may compound this problem with the risk of thinning of the bones too (osteoporosis). To reduce the risk of osteoporosis, ensure you are taking in enough calcium through your diet and, in the UK, taking supplemental vitamin D through the winter months as recommended, limiting alcohol, ensuring a healthy weight and diet, avoiding smoking and ensuring weight-bearing exercises are included in your exercise programme.
- Low levels of vitamin B12 due to poorer absorption from the bowel post radiotherapy.

Please let your health professional know if you are struggling with any of these side effects as further investigations and management may be necessary.

Chemotherapy

Chemotherapy is a treatment used to kill cancer cells by stopping them dividing, growing and spreading through the body. This can be used on its own or in combination with other treatments. Chemotherapy drugs can be very different and vary from cancer to cancer, and the choice can also be dependent on the stage of the cancer. This means the side-effect profiles will differ too.

Not everyone who has CRC requires chemotherapy, especially if you are diagnosed with stage 1 cancer. Very rarely, stage 2 cancer patients may need chemo, yet the majority with stage 3 cancer will require it. If the cancer is stage 4, chemotherapy may be used as part of a treatment plan.

What drugs are available?

The most common drugs used are:

- Capecitabine (Xeloda)
- Fluorouracil (5FU) often given with folinic acid (leucovorin)
- Oxaliplatin (Eloxatin)
- Irinotecan (Campto)
- Trifluridine and tipiracil (Lonsurf).
- Raltitexed (Tomudex) – usually reserved for those who are unable to have capecitabine, 5FU and oxaliplatin.

Often two or more drugs are given in combination. These are the most common combinations used:

- FOLFOX (folinic acid + fluorouracil + oxaliplatin)
- FOLFIRI (folinic acid + fluorouracil + irinotecan)
- CAPOX or XELOX (capecitabine + oxaliplatin) – the combination of chemotherapy I received
- FOLFOXIRI (folinic acid + fluorouracil + irinotecan + oxaliplatin)

Most chemotherapy agents are given through a vein intravenously, except capecitabine which is in tablet form. All the methods of gaining access to your veins to administer chemotherapy are listed below.

Ways to access veins to give chemotherapy intravenously

Cannula

A small thin plastic hollow tube is inserted into the back of your hand or your arm. The drip can then be attached to the cannula for the drugs to flow freely. The problem with this is that chemotherapy can be quite an irritant to the smaller veins so a situation where you 'run out' of veins may occur. For prolonged courses of chemo, a more central access is required to administer chemo through the larger diameter veins.

PICC line (peripherally inserted central catheter)

A PICC line is usually inserted in your upper arm above the elbow. It is a longer cannula and it is inserted with local anaesthetic. It stays in place for the duration of treatment and bloods can be taken from it as well. They are flushed weekly. They can catch, so it's important to keep them secure, and they usually have a waterproof dressing which is changed weekly. PICC line covers are also available.

Portacath

This involves a minor operation (I had mine with sedation and local anaesthetic). A port sits just under the skin on the left of your chest wall. The port has to be accessed during treatment with a needle, so a local anaesthetic or 'numbing' cream is applied 30 minutes before the port needs to be accessed. This will be removed once all treatment has finished.

These access sites can become infected so make sure you seek medical help if you have a fever, develop redness, pain or swelling around the area or pus leaks out. PICC and port lines also have a risk of blood clots forming in the vein. Symptoms include redness, swelling or tenderness of the arm, chest area or into the neck, a swollen hand on the side of the PICC line or shortness of breath. Again, please seek help from your oncology team in the event of any of these symptoms.

Drugs are often given in cycles and these can vary in length from one to four weeks depending on the drug concoction you are given.

You will be given information about each agent and regime and ways to manage side effects from your oncology team and I will discuss some of these in more detail shortly.

How did I feel having chemotherapy which I received after surgery as an adjuvant therapy?

Being told I needed chemotherapy was just a given. I'd already been spared chemo-radiotherapy prior to my cancer surgery and I knew from the outset there would be no escaping chemotherapy after. I would take whatever treatment my oncologist threw at me, including the kitchen sink, to reduce my chance of recurrence. As fewer lymph nodes were involved than initially thought, it was felt on balance, the duration of chemotherapy I would need could be reduced from six months to three months. This equated to four cycles every three weeks of oxaliplatin (an infusion through my port in the chemotherapy suite) and capecitabine tablets for two weeks, with a week off chemotherapy to recuperate in between. These drug-free weeks were a salvation from the mental and physical effects of chemotherapy. Patterns emerged of side effects and my ability to function, and I learnt when to plan for exercise and fun trips out with family, friends and the children, where I saw a piece of the old me, as did others.

The first thing to remember is that everyone reacts to treatment and treatment regimes differently. As mentioned, keep a diary, not just to share with your specialist so you can hopefully manage the side effects better, but also for you so you know what to expect and can prepare yourself for each cycle. This could include ensuring you have gloves for cold-induced peripheral neuropathy, or keeping a vomit bowl by your side, or your favourite foods in stock if you don't feel like eating the first few days after chemo. A pattern evolves and those around you tune into the frequency as well. I know my children began to see a pattern of when 'mummy was around and present' to just not seeing her really for the first week of each cycle. When I was in my treatment-free week of a three-weekly cycle, their mummy would 'return', and as it came to the end of that week, they would also fear the next cycle.

Starting chemotherapy was fuelled with anxiety and anticipation, with no idea what would be coming next. It was only when I realized how chemo did affect me during the first cycle that I started to dread the next one, knowing what havoc would occur once more.

I struggled with chemo, I won't lie. Not everyone struggles as much as I did. I left little time for physical or mental recovery between surgeries before throwing myself into chemo and I also tend to be super-sensitive to any drugs, even those taken previously for minor ailments, in comparison to others.

What side effects can I expect from chemotherapy?

Many of the symptoms can be controlled by giving medications to counteract the side effects but it is a balancing act, and a diary of your symptoms helps your oncologist tweak drugs and add in others to combat side effects as needed. This is in the hope you can complete and tolerate the cycles of chemotherapy offered with the least side effects. Side effects are also cumulative. This means you may feel reasonable the first few cycles but as time goes on, these side effects build up and can increase.

Below, I have listed a variety of general side effects one may experience with chemotherapy, often with more anecdotes from the times I was going through treatment and some self-help along the way.

Diarrhoea – 'Someone please send help!'

Many chemotherapy agents cause diarrhoea. The symptoms tend to be worse following bowel surgery when part of the colon or rectum is removed. A lot of the advice below will seem counterintuitive to having a healthy diet during chemo but remember this is short term and people can become quite unwell if the diarrhoea is severe.

Tips: How to help reduce diarrhoea during chemo

- Drink plenty of water.
- Reduce insoluble fibres (low-irritant, high-fibre diet – see Useful Resources).
- Avoid fizzy or alcoholic drinks.
- Avoid spicy food, pulses (beans and lentils) and deep-fried food.
- Stop laxatives.
- Limit lactose products or milk to see if this improves symptoms.
- Use antidiarrhoeal medications (e.g. loperamide tablets or liquid preferable (if stoma or frequent bowel movements).
- Skin protection for the bottom/anus area.
- If the diarrhoea episodes are frequent (>6 times in 24 hours), or associated with blood in the stool, inability to drink fluids, or you are experiencing severe pain, please contact your hospital team or oncology specialist nurse.

Feeling sick (nausea) and vomiting – 'Fetch me a bucket NOW!'

Chemotherapy can make you feel sick which can reduce your appetite and desire to eat. As a doctor, advice during chemo is to try to maintain a healthy diet. From my own experience as a patient, this wasn't always possible and for one week of each cycle, I would live off beige food on repeat, my repertoire including cheese toasties, rich tea biscuits, scones with no raisins and rice crispies. If this is you, do not beat yourself up over it, as my dietary repertoire would broaden once the nausea passed and I made a conscious effort to try to eat a more balanced meal. Some people find that eating small amounts of food at regular intervals can also help control the feelings of nausea. Eating something before taking capecitabine tablets or something with ginger in, such as tea, may help reduce nausea too. My advice is eat what you can, it's far better than not eating at all.

Vomiting is less common. Anti-sickness tablets are often given with chemotherapy. However, if you vomit more than once in any 24-hour period or can't keep food or drink down, it's important to contact your oncology helpline to discuss alternative options.

Tiredness and weakness (fatigue)

Fatigue can occur during and after treatment. This symptom has a dedicated chapter (see Chapter 11) as it is one that is multifactorial and deserves a lengthier discussion.

Increased risk of infection

The chemotherapy also affects your blood cells, including your infection-fighting cells, or white bloods cells, specifically your neutrophils. This can result in low levels of neutrophils, called neutropaenia. You will be asked to monitor your temperature and if it spikes above 38 degrees, or you feel unwell, it is important to contact your specialist team as soon as possible, or your oncology treatment hotline, and it is likely you will need to go to hospital for further assessment. Hygiene measures are also important, including hand washing and avoiding those with active infection. It is also sensible to avoid foods that may carry bacteria such as unpasteurized cheeses, honey and so on.

Symptoms of an infection include:

- Feeling shivery and shaking
- Sore throat
- Cough
- Breathlessness
- Diarrhoea
- Needing to pass urine (pee) a lot, or discomfort when you pass urine.

Bruising and bleeding

You may be more prone to bruising and bleeding – such as nose bleeds, gum bleeds, heavier periods, and tiny red or purple spots in your skin or blood in your urine or poo. This is because chemotherapy can reduce the number of platelets in your blood which help blood clot. These again should be monitored with each cycle.

Anaemia

Chemotherapy can reduce the number of red blood cells in your blood resulting in anaemia. Red blood cells carry oxygen around the body. You may have symptoms such as pale skin, a lack of energy, feeling breathless or dizzy and light-headed.

Brain fog or chemo brain – 'Sorry, what's my name again?'

Medically known as 'cancer-related cognitive dysfunction or impairment', it has been reported that 45–78 per cent of cancer patients are affected. I found it unbelievably frustrating and embarrassing. The mental fog and cognitive dysfunction. The chemo brain. I would forget names. Some weeks, I re-named half of my closest friends and family. When checking in to see my oncologist one time, I briefly forgot my own! I would lose my train of thought, freezing mid-sentence, and mind blank, looking lost and spaced out, a brief period of absence. And I would have such trouble word-finding. Writing my Instagram posts became more taxing, my mind drawing blanks. Once a professional multi-tasker, completing single tasks without distraction became an enormous challenge, everything taking so much longer! My usual organized chaos was, frankly, disorganized. I spent much of my time subjecting my wonderful friends and family to multiple renditions of the same anecdotes, to which they already knew the punchline!

I had a stack of magazines, periodicals and books awaiting my attention, but I couldn't focus on them. I constantly misplaced things, too – keys, wallet, glasses, shoes … (no change there, my husband tells me!). I would also like to add here a huge debt of thanks to the inventor of the 'Find my phone' app: you are a wonderful human being; I lost count of how many times my phone took its leave of me!

I know this was all to be expected, but the list of symptoms below and the effect they had left me feeling overwhelmed, and at times, simply lost. Below is a list of the symptoms individuals may experience with chemo brain:

- Brain fog
- Inability to concentrate
- Memory problems and forgetfulness, unable to keep track of names, dates, items
- Difficulty finding the right word – 'where are my ... keys ... I mean, sunglasses?'
- Finding it hard to learn new things
- Easily distracted
- Feeling spaced out
- Disorganized
- Taking longer than normal to complete tasks.

So, why does it happen?

It is multifactorial – a cocktail of drug therapies, surgical intervention and recovery, ongoing chemotherapy, radiotherapy, hormonal treatments, the cancer, the intense emotion, incalculable amount of stress and anxiety, poor nutritional intake, transient/permanent/acute-onset menopause, intercurrent infection, fluctuating levels of pain, myriad side effects, cumulative and inexorable fatigue, constant sleep deprivation, hormonal disturbances ... and the mixture can be very debilitating in a completely different way to the physical symptoms. In my experience, the severity and consequences would vary day to day depending on what else I was dealing with that day.

Explaining how you feel to loved ones can be really insightful and help them understand how they can help make things easier for you.

How could you help, should we meet on the street?

This is what I would have divulged to someone who came across me while I was on chemo. 'If I repeat myself, please tell me. If I forget things I really should know, please remind me. If my concentration has lapsed and I'm looking vaguely into the distance, I'm not intentionally being impolite, so please bear with me. And when I'm emotional, or irrational, out of character, or out of sorts, you just being there, trying to understand, is more than plenty.'

The single best piece of advice I can offer is this. Try to keep life simple, and go easy on yourself.

- Try to complete tasks when you are at your best.
- Play games or do puzzles, Sudoku, crosswords.
- Exercise and get some fresh air.
- Try to follow a healthy diet.
- Practise good sleep hygiene.
- Get plenty of rest and relaxation, not always achievable, I know. However, reducing stress is really beneficial.
- Write lists ... lots of them. (And then never get round to them till days later because you forgot you wrote a list.)
- Take photos ...
- ... and a second pair of ears to your hospital appointments, or you can ask your team if you can record the consult so you can listen to it afterwards.

This will improve after treatment ends ... slowly. Patients report that symptoms continue to improve up to six months after the point that treatment has ended.

Chemo rage – 'Will you please just get out of my sight?'

Definition by Google: 'a completely reasonable response to cancer and the many difficulties it brings. But for some people, their cancer treatment is accompanied by a sudden, uncharacteristic increase in irritability, angry outbursts, and even aggressive behaviour.'

This. It made me feel as if I was possessed at times. It seemed more noticeable as the cycles progressed and my personal belief was that it was steroid-related (used for anti-sickness). Looking back there was more than one factor: drugs were causative, but so was the stress of the situation, the helplessness, the frustration, the sleep deprivation and absolute fatigue. Chemo rage seemed to rear its ugly head towards the end of the day. I developed an acute intolerance to noise and chaos – tricky with a six- and seven-year-old in the house – and I felt extremely impatient. Tolerance levels were at an all-time low. I'll admit one day I wanted to take a crow bar to my house and smash everything up in pure frustration at being housebound, ill and in a pretty bad place. But thankfully that, too, did pass quickly.

Having insight into this emotion is quite upsetting. It's raw and comes from nowhere, sometimes when you least expect it. It's intense. Very intense. But so very irrational. So, what could I do apart from wait for the drugs to come out of my system?

Well, firstly, I bought ear defenders! Initially I was dubious, however they were extremely useful. I explained to the children that 'the medicines make mummy more sensitive to noise'. I could still hear them and communicate, but everything was quieter. I also found it helped with the drug-induced migraines, too, when noise hypersensitivity was also present. I would try to walk away from whatever I was doing if I felt the red sea of rage come crashing in. And importantly, I said 'sorry' ... a lot, because this wasn't really me.

The good news is that chemo rage doesn't affect everyone and should settle very quickly once you come off the medication and chemotherapy.

Heightened senses – 'Your breath stinks!'

Not only did chemo cause noise intolerance, but my sense of smell resembled that of a bloodhound. Hyperosmia (heightened sense of smell) or dysosmia (a distorted perception of smell) can affect up to 40 per cent of patients on chemo. Most smells would precipitate nausea and make my stomach turn.

Aftershave, perfumes, soap, food, people, even myself! I felt I could smell the chemo oozing out of my pores at times, on my bedclothes, bed linen, urine – it was vile and even washing didn't seem to eliminate the odour at times. It's a chemically foul smell that my husband never seemed to notice. I momentarily thought about spraying myself with air freshener although I think that would have set me off too. It's all to do with the metabolites from the chemo being excreted through bodily fluids and the change in natural bacteria flora on the skin whilst on chemo.

I remember distinctly in cycle one daily telling my poor, tolerant husband that he stank and he ended up asking the children, and a colleague at work, to reassure him that he didn't and that the problem lay with me! Again this settles once you are off the chemotherapy.

The mouth

Since we are going through the senses and the effects of cancer upon them, how could we leave out taste? Reduced taste (hypogeusia), loss of taste (ageusia) and altered taste (dysgeusia) are the main disturbances to taste. For some patients this can lead to weight loss and malnutrition. Certain chemotherapy agents obliterate cells in your oral cavity and it's safe to say chemo temporarily changed my sense of taste, too. Being a food lover, my taste buds were less than impressed. Food seemed bland and often tasted bitter, with a metallic taste (which tends to be from the oxaliplatin – as it's a platinum-containing drug, for all of us with expensive tastes!). And the pleasure of eating diminished. I never knew quite what I fancied. Strong flavours were paramount so we used plenty of spices, herbs and marinades. I ate or drank citrus produce which cleanses the taste buds, but avoid at all costs if you have stomatitis (inflammation of the lining of the mouth causing soreness).

Others find that food can taste very sweet. Many crave sugary foods and some develop a sudden dislike to a food. For me, sadly, this was avocado, which conversely I was eating daily before chemo while I had a stoma.

Thankfully, recovery of the taste buds only takes a few weeks after chemo finishes and, believe me, I savoured the taste of every mouthful when it returned, as well as many avocados!

Appetite, weight changes and diet

I'm leaving this extract here below that I wrote during treatment. We are always told to eat well, be healthy, keep hydrated, but it was far from easy to follow these simple rules when in treatment. As a doctor, this was really insightful, as my job involves giving out lifestyle advice that seemingly should be straightforward, but can be so complex on so many levels.

Pre-chemotherapy checkup – cycle 2

They call my name. I'm led to the scales. I hold my breath.

Yes!!! I've passed the test. I'm exactly the same weight, which is great because I lost weight in week 1 due to persistent nausea, lack of appetite and change in taste caused by my chemo. Every time I attend hospital, I feel as if I'm checking in for WeightWatchers, as I'm led to the scales on check-in, but the aim is not to lose weight! As someone who never weighs themselves, it is rather foreign and something that for some reason just doesn't sit right with me. However, I've now managed to put weight back on by eating foods I would not usually overindulge in on weeks 2 and 3.

My diet is far from what it would be normally, with the dietary limitations imposed post-stoma reversal and bowel surgery (essentially avoid onions, pulses, and a low-residue diet avoiding raw vegetables, high insoluble fibre foods and foods with strings, pips, seeds and skin). And I'll be honest – I've really struggled with this. I also crave carbs and don't fancy protein as much, although my medical brain keeps telling me I need protein for cell repair and to keep up my muscle mass as I am obliterated by chemo. Some days I just don't think I'm getting the nutrients I need in to me. And that used to stress me out. But I'm trying to stay focused that this is (hopefully) short term.

Stereotypically patients on chemo are thought to lose weight, but many gain weight through chemo too. Inactivity, side effects of steroids, and so forth all contribute. My oncologist wants me to maintain mine for now.

With the above in mind, I'm sent to the cancer specialist dietician, with my brother as my second pair of ears. It was fantastically informative, and I'm now armed with the do's and dont's to see me through.

Hair loss

When I was told initially that I needed chemo, I was all set to buy a wig before treatment started. However, unlike many other chemotherapy agents, total hair loss is not common with the XELOX/FOLFOX regimes. Hair loss usually starts two to three weeks after treatment starts. I've always had long hair, and decided to change my mane on the advice of a hairdresser pre chemo to a shorter, more layered style.

I was fortunate to have quite thick hair to start with so people keep telling me 'you haven't lost any hair', but I knew it was thinning. There was often a rug of hair left in the bed in the morning, and a fur ball in my hairbrush.

Initially this was upsetting as it was a constant reminder of cancer, but now I know how lucky I am to still have a lot of my hair left.

Tips: To help minimize hair loss and thinning
- Cut hair shorter and add more layers to add volume.
- Avoid extensions/Brazilian blow dry/any chemical treatments – all these will weaken the hair.
- Don't brush it too often. In fact some days, I avoided it altogether. Use a baby brush as it is gentler.
- Avoid washing hair frequently.

- Avoid products, hairdryers, straighteners.
- Avoid tight hairstyles and wear a hair net in bed.
- Avoid dying your hair while having chemo. Chemo has definitely gifted me some new grey hairs!
- Use paraben-free shampoo/conditioner and 0 ph products.
- No eyelash extensions during, or six months after, treatment.

If you do experience total hair loss with treatment, there are some wonderful wig companies and head scarves out there that may help your confidence and the way you feel about yourself.

Drug-specific side effects

Moving on from general side effects caused by chemotherapy, we know that each individual drug often has its own drug-specific side effects and some of these are listed below for each drug.

Oxaliplatin Cold Dysaesthesias and Chemotherapy Induced Peripheral Neuropathy (CIPN)

Oxaliplatin Cold dysaesthesia refers to an unusual side effect causing an increased sensitivity of certain body parts to the cold. Symptoms are usually severe after the infusion and subsequently wane, but can increase in severity with each cycle. CIPN is a condition caused by a range of chemotherapy agents including oxaliplatin, which causes nerve damage that may be progressive and for some irreversible and triggered by the cold. It usually manifests as numbness, more often than pain. The severity varies from patient to patient, and below I share my experience of these conditions from my journal:

I never knew a salt and vinegar crisp could inflict so much pain! I was watching my first drip of oxaliplatin run through my port in my chest, and had settled in for the lengthy chemo session ahead. Drip. Drip. Drip. My husband and I had overcome the shock of having my port being accessed and the difficulties they had with that, and we came prepared with plenty of snacks for the day. As my husband offered me a crisp, I took a bite and I was not prepared for what came next. One can only describe a searing electric pain radiating through my throat, to my jaw and to my ears with the sensation that my throat was closing up. It was truly bizarre but my contorted facial expressions saw my husband burst out in nervous laughter as we were both unsure what was going on. I was then offered a bite of a sandwich ... No, no no ... in fact this made things worse, the cold filling magnified the sensation, but thankfully after a few seconds, it passed. Later, we realized it was a side effect of oxaliplatin called laryngeal dysaesthesia (usually cold induced – causing throat spasm or tightness, pins and needles, pains radiating into the jaw … you get the picture). Never did cold food or drink pass my lips again, until one week after my infusion was securely under my belt, where cold water could pass my lips once more and these symptoms passed.

After I was disconnected from the chemotherapy, I left the hospital with my twice daily tablet chemotherapy (capecitabine), high-dose steroids and anti-sickness meds looking utterly ridiculous – ski-gloves, woolly hat, blanket scarf wrapped round my face, AND woolly boots. I'd been warned about the cold-induced neuropathy so I came armed to try to avoid the cold air which can precipitate electric shock like pains or pins and needles in my hands, feet and throat. I felt smug as I felt well prepared, however as a gust of wind blew past, all I could feel were daggers piercing through my eyes. I wrapped the scarf round my face to take shelter and my husband guided me to the car, where I turned the heating onto full blast.

When we reached home, I was exhausted and I took my woolly protective boots off and as soon as my feet touched our wooden floor, the burning started once more. I clambered into the bedroom to find a second pair of thick socks, and as I touched the cold metal handle to open the drawer, it triggered pains in my fingers once more. So I chose to leave my gloves on and eat dinner with a plastic spoon. Oven gloves when opening the fridge probably won't be overkill. Today I learnt a lot … TOUCH NOTHING COLD. I'll be even more prepared next time.

During this time hand warmers and thermals became my best friends, and I never left the house without gloves and thermal socks. No cold drinks. No cold knives and forks. In fact, a kind friend had acknowledged my inability to use cutlery and bought me an extremely practical bamboo set. The thoughtfulness of humans during my illness was unreal.

For me, the neuropathy was acute whilst on treatment. It was quite something else. Severe leg cramps on day one to the point I couldn't walk. More comedy moments rolled in, as my husband lovingly tried to carry me to the bathroom as I couldn't walk due to the pain, and then ending up with a head injury as he misjudged the door frame to the bathroom. Thankfully the cramps only lasted 24 hours.

What can I do about CIPN?

Unfortunately, CIPN affects about 60 per cent of patients and is a common reason for a dose reduction or for treatment actually being stopped. My dose after the first cycle was certainly reduced for this reason. The severity worsens as each cycle passes. It's important to try to avoid the cold and use protection to mitigate the number of attacks to the nerves.

Up to half of patients can experience a degree of symptoms post treatment. It may appear to settle when treatment ends, but it can present later on. In fact it can come back up to a year after treatment is completed. A small percentage of patients can have irreversible damage, therefore it is very important they are honest at each consultation about how much they are affected, to try to prevent long-term damage.

Through treatment, I was given high-dose pyridoxine (a vitamin B supplement). Evidence is contradictory – some studies show benefit, some don't, but as it is a harmless supplement, some oncologists use it. In my clinical experience, nerves need time to regenerate, a year to 18 months, but it has been documented that symptoms, especially caused by oxaliplatin, can last the longest out of the chemotherapy drugs, sometimes up to six years. On the plus side, if the drugs had this effect on my nerves, just think what they've done to any pesky cancer cells lurking around. Here's hoping.

Unfortunately, there is little in terms of treatment for CIPN. Many medications have been evaluated. The only treatment that has been proven to reduce pain is duloxetine (it has multiple uses – depression, bladder problems, pain management). Dr Stewart suggests a TENS machine or painkillers such as tapentadol or gabapentin could be used to manage the pain too. However, I seemed to manage without and continued to take high dose pyridoxine for several months.

Someone had suggested to me a trial of acupuncture. Although there are no randomized controlled trials for this, there is some weak evidence to show it can help. I was willing to at least give this a go. I cannot be sure if it helped, or it was the passage of time, but I found having acupuncture an incredibly relaxing therapy in itself, channeling my inner calm. Hyperbaric Oxygen Therapy (HBOT) has also been used for neuropathy, although there is no strong evidence base currently. The hypothesis is this – by driving oxygen deep into tissues, it reduces cell death and pain symptoms. Hyperbaric oxygen potentially also stimulates the growth of new blood vessels, enabling the body to increase effective oxygen and nutrient delivery.

How am I now? I can safely say that the neuropathy has improved year on year. Four years on and I finally don't have to wear bed socks or slippers in the house all the time on our stone kitchen floor in the summer but they are firmly back on in the winter. I can touch frozen products or cold items for seconds rather than not at all. I have had to almost retrain my brain to talk to my hands and improve my co-ordination. I would struggle catching a tennis ball, for example, when I decided to take tennis lessons after treatment and felt clumsy, dropping things all the time, as the sensation in my hands had altered. It has still left me feeling relatively clumsy with my hands. Let's just say I won't be taking up a job in a bar soon!

Meet Claire, who recently started this treatment in combination with targeted therapy (see Chapter 9), for her stage 4 bowel cancer.

Claire (@fairyuss)

I'm now on treatment – irinotecan, folinic acid, fluorouracil (5-FU) and avastin. This time round, because I'm poorly and in pain, it's far more brutal and the side effects are greater. Lots of nausea, tiredness, tummy cramps, shivers and sniffles, headaches and moody days (which isn't me at all). And the weight loss has been frightening. I remind myself the side effects always ease and as you go through the cycles you get to know what to expect which gives confidence it's going to get better and you will feel better.

Fluorouracil (5-FU)

This remains the most widely used agent for colorectal cancer. Capecitabine is a 5-FU pro-drug developed to mimic the continuous infusion of 5-FU while avoiding the difficulties of a continuous intravenous administration via a pump over a few days at home. Both are equally effective and your specialist will decide which agent will suit your treatment regime better depending on what other drugs are being used.

One of the side effects specific to 5-FU is its impact on heart function, and some patients with heart conditions will not be able to have 5-FU and will need an alternative such as Raltitrexed. Therefore tests need to be carried out to check heart function and structure prior to, during and after treatment. DPD testing also needs to be carried out as it does with capecitabine (see above).

Rarely (less than 1 in 100 cases) someone taking 5-FU may suffer a heart attack or heart failure. Hence it is important to be aware if you have any of the following symptoms during or after treatment. Call your specialist team immediately if your symptoms include:

- Chest pain or tightness
- Breathlessness
- Palpitations or changes to your heartbeat.

Irinotecan (campto) – acute cholinergic syndrome

This chemotherapy can cause a rare side effect called 'acute cholinergic syndrome'. It can affect part of your nervous system that controls bodily secretions, and usually starts within 24 hours of taking the drug. Symptoms include profuse diarrhoea, stomach pains, runny nose, flushing, watering eyes, sweating profusely and excess saliva production. If you have any of those symptoms that start WITHIN 24 hours of taking this chemo, please let your specialist know immediately.

Toxicity vs efficacy

> After I saw my oncologist yesterday with my diary of never-ending side effects and an account of the last few weeks in cycle 1, she discussed reducing the doses of BOTH drugs by 10 per cent (oxaliplatin and capecitabine) as she felt I sounded as though I was suffering from toxicity from the drugs. Arghhhh! And my medic vs patient arguments start in my head. What if she reduces the dose and it loses its efficacy? I just need to get on with it surely and take the hit? But then what if chemo is stopped early again? Thankfully we had a long chat about toxicity and efficacy and we agreed that both of us would like me to be able to sit up for Christmas dinner! She has also given me a battery of drugs to counteract the increase in headaches and migraines (daily sumatriptan and propranolol), which can happen with chemo. Vitamin B6 50 mg three times a day to try to prevent oxaliplatin-induced neurotoxicity (damage to nerves). I've been on a lesser dose till now. She also advised laxatives day one and two to counteract the constipation from the ondansetron (anti-sickness) but Imodium later in the cycle for diarrhoea – it is extremely constipating stuff. She also referred me to a dietician. And so I'm armed with my supplies, ready for another cycle.

One final word regarding chemotherapy. The balancing act between toxicity (i.e. you feeling unwell on chemo with multiple side effects) and efficacy (how well the chemo will mop up or kill any cancer cells remaining) is a delicate balance and one I struggled at times to wrap my medical brain around. What if this lowered dose was not enough to kill any cancer cells left wandering? These are questions that have no right answers and your oncologist's aim will be to see you through many cycles of chemotherapy with the minimal number of side effects and toxicity. To reassure me, Dr Stewart discussed with me how the oncologist will choose the chemotherapy dose by the most toxic dose tolerated, not the minimum effective dose, therefore lowering doses is still likely to be effective. The relief!

Regardless of what chemotherapy agent or agents are being taken, it is really important to document side effects and let your team know if any occur as this needs to be managed, drug doses reviewed and as many cycles completed whilst trying to maintain some sort of quality of life at the same time. It's not easy, but with the right support, help and monitoring along the way, the impossible can seem possible.

8

Stage 4 cancer

Living with advanced colorectal cancer

Advanced bowel cancer, secondary CRC, metastatic CRC and stage 4 colorectal cancer are all interchangeable names given when cancer which has spread from the bowel to other organs in the body. Cancer cells break away from the primary tumour (in the bowel) and can spread and travel to another part of the body via the blood stream or lymphatic system. This cancer deposit is called a secondary tumour, or metastasis.

The most common places for bowel cancer to spread are:

- Liver
- Lungs
- Peritoneum (a thin layer of tissue that covers the organs in your tummy)
- Rarely, it can also spread to the bone, brain and ovaries (called a Krukenberg tumour).

Treating advanced bowel cancer

Deciding which treatment is best for metastatic colorectal cancer is complex as there are so many variables, listed below. These might include:

- Tumour size and the number of tumours
- Which organs are affected
- Whether there are any specific genetic mutations
- What treatments have already been given
- How fit and healthy the patient is – how much treatment they can tolerate
- How they have responded to other treatment so far
- The side effects of treatment and ability of the patient to tolerate them.

Your doctor or clinical nurse specialist will talk you through the benefits and possible risks and answer any questions you may have. Once you are fully informed, your healthcare team will help you make a decision on which treatment is best for you.

Treatment for advanced bowel cancer can include:

- Surgery
- Chemotherapy
- Radiotherapy
- Targeted therapy or immunotherapy (see Chapter 9).

Some treatments are specific to the part of the body that the cancer has spread to. The type of treatment you have will depend upon the aim of the treatment. The aim could be:

- To remove the tumour completely, with the intent to be cancer-free.
- To shrink the tumour, so that in some cases, it might be possible to remove it at a later stage.
- To keep the cancer under control. This is a type of palliative care that aims to prolong and improve quality of life and to help you remain active for as long as possible. You may have palliative care for several years. It can also be referred to as supportive care. Some patients have such good responses to palliative treatment that the cancer can be removed.
- To help manage the symptoms of bowel cancer, reduce the side effects of treatment and improve your quality of life. This is a type of palliative care that is sometimes called end-of-life care. The change to end-of-life care is gradual and your healthcare team will support you in deciding how to continue your treatment.

Treatment plans can be complicated and can change, which can be disconcerting, ever readjusting your own sails. Between treatments it can be useful to see how you are feeling, what has been achieved and to think about the next steps. Speak to your healthcare team if you have any questions or concerns about your treatment, symptoms or side effects.

Bowel cancer that has spread to the lungs

It's important to be aware of the signs and symptoms that could indicate spread to the lungs (see Chapter 14), and it is important to get checked. Most of the time, there may be another explanation that is not cancer related. If you are under routine surveillance, CT scans may also pick up cancer that has spread to the lungs; you may have no symptoms and be completely unaware.

There are a number of treatment modalities available for spread to the lungs, and I have outlined them below. Further information regarding all these therapies can be found on Bowel Cancer UK or Cancer Research UK's websites (see Useful Resources).

1 Chemotherapy
2 Targeted therapy
3 Lung surgery
4 Ablative surgeries – radiofrequency ablation, cryoablation, microwave ablation
5 Stereotactic ablative body radiotherapy (SABR).

Lung surgery

Surgery is often carried out in specialist centres. This may be an option straight off as a first line or after you have had another type of treatment first, for example chemotherapy. Types of lung surgery available include:

• Wedge resection – for tumours near the outer edge
• Lobectomy
• Segmentectomy – for the removal of larger tumours or tumours in the middle of the lung.

If your cancer has spread to both lungs, one lung will be treated at a time, often with a combination of treatments. Surgery can be via a keyhole approach (laparoscopic) or if it is not possible to remove the cancer by keyhole surgery, you may need to have open surgery. This is also called a thoracotomy.

Surgery is not suitable for all so do explore your options with your specialist team. Some of these techniques are described below.

Ablative therapies

Cancer cells are destroyed by applying various energy waves through probes placed on to your skin or during surgery. You may have local anaesthetic or general anaesthetic depending on the procedure.

Treatment is guided by ultrasound or CT scans. There are various different techniques of ablative therapy that can used as outlined below.

Radiofrequency ablation (RFA)

Cancer cells are destroyed by using the heat from radio waves. This can completely remove all the cancerous cells, shrink down the tumour or control symptoms.

Microwave ablation

Cancer cells are destroyed by heat generated by microwaves emitted from a probe. If your tumour is sizeable, or close to important structures such as blood vessels, they may suggest this method of treatment.

Cryoablation

Cancer cells are destroyed by freezing the tumour. The frozen tumour is then defrosted for fifteen minutes and then refrozen multiple times.

Stereotactic ablative body radiotherapy (SABR)

This is a type of external radiotherapy, available in specialist centres. It destroys cancer in specific areas using radiotherapy.

CyberKnife is one form of SABR. High-dose radiotherapy is concentrated onto the cancer by thin beams of radiation which target the cancer specifically, from numerous directions.

Bowel cancer that has spread to the liver

After spread to the lymph nodes, the liver is the next most common site for CRC spread to occur. Advancing techniques have seen survival rates increase over the years in those where there has been spread to the liver.

What would I expect to feel if the cancer had spread to my liver?

You may experience some of the symptoms one would find with colorectal cancer: tiredness, low energy levels, and a lack of appetite. However, specific symptoms include those listed in Chapter 14. For this reason, it is important that if you have any unusual symptoms, you let a health professional know, be it your doctor or cancer team. On the converse, you may not experience any symptoms at all, and the tumour may be picked up on routine surveillance CT scans.

Meet Emma, aged 36. She found out that she had a liver cancer recurrence after initially having been given the all-clear in September 2020.

Emma (emma_campbell_84)

I was due a regular surveillance scan when I was away, but I pushed it back to February 2022, because I had just come back from a trip climbing Mount Kilimanjaro. I returned to a CT scan letter. I still felt fine, and had been with no evidence of disease since my bowel op in September 2020, so for around a year and a half, with no additional treatment or medication at all, so I was feeling ok about it. But like any scan, no matter what the situation, you have scanxiety, the fear of 'what if these results don't show what I want them to...?'. Despite just summiting Kilimanjaro, and feeling great, about a week after the scan, I received a call. My surgeon wanted to see me the next day... it didn't sound good. We tried different scenarios around in our heads to explain why he wanted to see me so urgently... but our fears were confirmed and my cancer had indeed returned.

I didn't feel how I expected to when my surgeon told me the news. He is an amazing consultant and before we had a chance to even think about it, he sugar-coated the news that the cancer was back in my liver by immediately saying 'but it is small, it is in the same area as last time' and most importantly, 'it is treatable'. He had even been on the phone already to speak with the liver specialist so had a vague plan. This, coupled with the fact that I deep down always kind of knew that the cancer would return in the liver (because I hadn't had liver surgery the first time), meant that news of a reoccurrence did not trigger the devastating emotions I thought it would. My husband was probably more shocked at the news than me and although obviously I did not want to hear it, somehow (and this is going to sound strange) it was almost a relief. A relief that what I kind of always knew would happen had now done so, and a relief that my reoccurrence was localized to the same place as before, one tiny met in the liver and nowhere else, and it was treatable. That's what I told myself, and that is the mindset I took to deal with the cancer coming back.

There are many options available to treat CRC that has spread to the liver, and treatment can be individualized.

1 Chemotherapy
2 Targeted therapy
3 Liver surgery – this may be an option straight off as a first line, or after you have had another type of treatment first, for example chemotherapy

4 Ablative surgeries – radiofrequency ablation

5 Embolization therapy

6 DEBIRI-TACE

7 Selective internal radiation therapy (SIRT)

Liver surgery

The liver is a wonderful organ in that it has a unique ability to regenerate after tissue has been removed. In fact, up to 50 per cent of the liver can be removed and it will still replenish itself! Removing secondary cancer in the liver can be very successful. Other treatment methods such as chemotherapy may be required before surgery.

Liver surgery is usually carried out in specialist liver cancer centres. The surgery may be keyhole or open.

Types of liver surgery (liver resection) include:

- Left hemihepatectomy – the surgeon removed up to half the liver containing the tumour on the left side.
- Right hemihepatectomy – the surgeon removed up to half the liver containing the tumour on the right side.
- Two-step hepatectomy procedures – if there are tumours on the right and left sides of the liver, a two-step procedure can be performed, when one operation follows another operation several weeks later to attend to the tumour on the other side. Surgery can be done again, via a keyhole or open approach, but it depends on the surgery required.

You may need to have treatment before surgery to shrink the tumour. This is called neoadjuvant therapy. It can include chemotherapy and other specialized techniques.

Some patients might have treatment to encourage healthy parts of their liver to grow before surgery. This is called a portal vein embolization. A needle is put into the stomach area (abdomen) and guided by x-ray to a blood vessel in your liver. You will have a local anaesthetic. The procedure takes about an hour and you will probably stay in hospital for one night.

Not everyone can have liver surgery due to a number of factors including size, location and the number of tumour deposits. If you can't have surgery there could be different treatment options that are suitable for you. Your healthcare team will discuss these with you, and I've outlined some of these below.

Ablative therapies

We looked at ablative therapies earlier – here are the ablative procedures that are used to destroy tumours in the liver.

- Radiofrequency ablation (RFA)
- Microwave ablation
- NanoKnife – irreversible electroporation (IRE)

NanoKnife is available in the USA, but not available in certain areas of the UK on the NHS, but can sometimes be given as part of a clinical trial. Cancer cells are destroyed by electrical pulses.

Stereotactic ablative radiotherapy (SABR)

This includes therapies such as CyberKnife TM – as discussed above.

High intensity frequency ultrasound (HIFU)

HIFU is a new and emerging treatment for liver cancer. The beauty is that it is non-invasive so has minimal side effects. Ultrasound beams containing high-energy ultrasound waves are targeted towards the tumour and heat it, thereby destroying it by thermal damage. There are centres conducting clinical trials with this technique, and you would need to ask your team for more details to see if you would be eligible. Studies have shown that it is safe, and there is an excellent response to this treatment and prognosis longer term.

Embolization treatment

Embolization treatments use very small beads to block (embolize) blood vessels so that less blood goes to a part of the liver. The beads are delivered to your liver through a catheter. They stop blood going to the tumour which means the cancer cells are starved and can be destroyed. You will have either a general or local anaesthetic as part of this procedure.

DEBIRI-TACE

Small beads loaded with the chemotherapy drug irinotecan are placed into the liver. The beads block the blood supply and deliver chemotherapy to the cancer. This procedure usually takes around one to two hours. After the procedure, you will usually stay in hospital overnight.

Selective internal radiation therapy (SIRT)

Tiny radioactive beads are inserted into a blood vessel (artery) in the liver. These beads block the artery, while simultaneously emitting radiation to the surrounding cancer cells, thereby destroying them. As the radiation dose not travel far, the rest of the tissue is spared.

Bowel cancer that has spread to the lining of the abdominal cavity (peritoneal metastasis)

Symptoms may include bloating, tummy swelling, tummy pain, indigestion, feeling full after eating, nausea and vomiting, loss of appetite, weight loss or a change in bowel habit.

Treatment may include chemotherapy, targeted therapy or surgery. There are also newer innovative technologies for treating cancer in the peritoneum, some of which may be available to you, for example HIPEC and PIPAC – if this is the case, your multidisciplinary team will decide an appropriate treatment plan for you, taking into account your personal situation.

The HIPEC (hyperthermic intraperitoneal chemotherapy) technique combines surgery with chemotherapy. First the surgeons carry out surgery to remove all the tumour deposits they can visualize on the lining of the abdomen (the peritoneum), or deposits on any organs such as the liver or stomach. At the end of surgery, a warmed dose of chemotherapy is administered into the abdominal cavity (the heat increases penetration of the chemotherapy into cells). This aims to mop up any cancer cells invisible to the naked eye.

PIPAC (pressurized intraperitoneal aerosol chemotherapy) involves a laparoscopic (keyhole) surgical approach. A special cannula is used to distribute the chemotherapy in the form of an aerosol or 'fine rain' directly reaching the areas affected by the tumour. It can be repeated every four to six weeks, with each patient having two or three treatments. Unlike HIPEC, if there are many tumours in the peritoneum, PIPAC can be used to try to reduce the number and size of tumours, reducing the cancer burden, which may allow HIPEC at a later date.

How do I live well with a stage 4 diagnosis?

What I've witnessed and learnt from the community I've entered is that, regardless of diagnosis, you can thrive with a stage 4 diagnosis. I asked Emma to talk to me about how she lives since receiving her stage 4 diagnosis, and here she speaks candidly about her own experience.

My team never told me (and still to this day haven't) what stage my cancer was. I subsequently worked it out: because the cancer had spread to another organ, it is classed as stage 4 cancer. I remember when I worked it out for myself, the feeling of my heart sinking so low it almost hit the floor. Alongside that I inadvertently read statistics around stage 4 bowel cancer and that day was the lowest I have ever felt. But that moment changed everything for me with my cancer journey, for the better. I would not be labelled as a stage – I still can't bear to say it out loud; I would not dwell on the percentages and the data, but instead chose to do the opposite. To be super positive to the point where I started to believe the words in my head, when I was telling myself I would be ok; I would get through this and not just survive it but thrive! That was such a powerful tool I can't begin to tell you. And because I took control so early on, it meant I had the power. If I described my cancer I would say 'advanced cancer' or 'bowel cancer with liver mets'. Although essentially the same thing, these ways of describing my diagnosis made me feel more comfortable, gave me the control I needed and allowed me to maintain a positive outlook. Never again would I let myself get into that dark place, when I felt my heart hit the floor. This is of course my personal coping strategy; many others I know will happily and proudly share their stage. But for me it just wasn't and still now isn't something I am comfortable talking about. (Writing this was so hard!) But you do whatever you need to do to cope; there's no rule book and like everything in life, we all deal with things differently.

I tried to embrace the new life I had been given, despite my fears of reoccurrence in the liver. And I lived my life … With regular scans, which still confirmed no evidence of cancer. I felt fine, I was living again and living differently; I was living big. I desperately wanted to show myself, to show my children and to show cancer itself that I was so much more than the disease which had become such as huge part of my existence. So what better way to say 'up yours, cancer' than to climb Mount Kilimanjaro in Africa, the world's tallest free standing mountain, and to do so for the charity Bowel Cancer UK. So that's what I did, alongside some other friends and bowel cancer survivors: just two years on from my diagnosis, still cancer free (or so I thought), in January 2022 we summited Kilimanjaro after a nine-day trek. It was one of the hardest things I have ever done, but also one of my proudest moments. And it really and truly felt like the biggest 'F you cancer' that we could have done.

Following on from Emma's positive outlook, I asked a number of other stage 4 thrivers about how they try to live well and thrive with a stage 4 diagnosis. These were some of their most common answers:

- Learn to accept your diagnosis. The anticipatory anxiety we spoke about earlier – the 'what ifs?' and 'why me's?' and 'if onlys' can become all-encompassing and the focus should be on the here and now and on treatment: what can be done about the situation, rather than dwelling on the problem itself. Adopting a growth mindset can help with this in terms of changing your outlook and thinking instead, 'What can I do to make the most of life right now?'

- Take each day at a time. Uncertainty with cancer is crippling at any stage, but with stage 4, it does hit hard. Finding a way to live in the moment and day to day, having short-term goals to see you through, using some of the tools we discussed in Chapter 16, can help facilitate 'living life' and thriving day to day.

- Try not to Google. I remember the wonderful Dame Deborah James saying, 'If you are diagnosed with a stage 4 cancer, the first thing you shouldn't do is Google it!' And I stand by her advice. A growing number of patients with stage 4 cancer are living longer with stage 4 and a small group, where spread is to the liver or lungs, for example, are cured. Googling 'stage 4 cancer' is not usually advisable, and if you have done so, you need to remember that survival rates are based on studies that were done a few years ago, in certain populations. With advances in treatment regimes, new studies are in progress as I write and the 'stats' will be ever-evolving. Treatment may be lifelong, so make sure you treat yourself along the way. Look at treatment as your life admin and lifeline, and try to fill your life with things you've always wanted to do when able to.

- Seek help and support from others. There is a stage 4 bowel cancer Facebook group and many other bowel cancer forums. Joining one for stage 4 cancer can be invaluable not only for support but to keep abreast of the latest research and treatments for this stage of disease. There are also online forums, for example on Bowel Cancer UK's website (see Useful Resources).

- Remember to live. Stage 4 can be that pivotal moment where actually you need to get busy living and doing all the things you want and are able to. Pity parties from time to time are absolutely ok as well as tears, anger, and all the emotions. Vent. Clear up and then, if you can, move on.

- New treatments are on the horizon, all the time. Stage 4 cancer patients are living longer than previously as a result. Are there any clinical trials you can enter? Many patients research this, or you could ask your specialists – remember, all the trials may have specific eligibility criteria so try to find out what these are to avoid disappointment.
- If you are unhappy with your treatment plan or feel you need a second opinion, advocate for yourself and ask for one.
- Maintain a healthy lifestyle, eat well, sleep, limit alcohol consumption, exercise, and stop smoking.
- Have hope – it can be hard, but sometimes that's all we have to hold on to.

Palliative care

Palliative care offers support, care and treatment for those with life-limiting illnesses. The care offered is holistic and takes into account the physical, emotional, psychological, social, and spiritual aspects of illness. The goal is to ensure the best possible quality of life. After you are diagnosed with stage 4 cancer, you can have the input of palliative care alongside active treatment. It is not simply for those who are imminently about to die or on end-of-life care. There is so much a palliative team can do.

I learnt first-hand about the fantastic service a hospice or palliative care team can offer, as I was fortunate enough through my GP training to work in a hospice for four months. What magical places they are. There is much heartache, but also much satisfaction when symptoms can be controlled, family can be supported, and an individual can have a dignified, peaceful and symptom-free death.

What can the palliative care team offer me?

- Pain management.
- Symptom control: improving the quality of life by controlling or reducing symptoms such as nausea, vomiting, appetite loss, diarrhoea, constipation, shortness of breath and so on.

- Mental health support – counselling or therapy.
- Support for you and your family – psychological, spiritual and social.
- Financial support.
- Assistance with living – helping arrange and co-ordinate care needed to help with the activities of daily life such as cooking, getting dressed and washed. Also recruiting input from physio-therapists for mobility issues, or an occupational therapist to make adjustments to the house, for example shower seats, stair lifts, commodes and so on.
- Help plan end-of-life care – if you are able to, think about your future and your end-of-life care decisions and wishes. Where would you like to die? At home, in hospital or in a hospice? What would your funeral arrangements be? This is extremely difficult, but it will help those around caring for you to know your specific wishes through their own time of distress.
- Bereavement or grief counselling.

Referrals to the palliative care team can be made through your doctor or the health professionals involved in your care.

End-of-life care

End-of-life care usually refers to the last year of life, and forms part of palliative care. Obviously no one has a crystal ball and the 'how long have I/they got left?' question that I've heard many times is not easy to answer: I've often been proven wrong. However, you may have been told that you will not get better, and that in fact you are approaching a life-limiting phase of end of life.

The purpose of end-of-life care is to ensure adequate symptom control, to allow the best quality of life possible, at that moment, and to maintain the patient's dignity throughout.

There is a wealth of support available for both the patient and their family (Useful Resources section) when it comes to end of life. This should offer support with the practicalities as well as the emotional aspects when it comes to this time.

Practicalities may involve decisions regarding where you may want to die (hospital, hospice or at home), from the funeral and arrangements, to administrative tasks and getting your affairs in order.

There will be a whole host of individuals potentially involved in your end-of-life care, including your family doctor, a palliative care team or hospice, plus other agencies such as physiotherapists, social workers, occupational therapists, complementary therapists, spiritual or religious leaders, counsellors, and specialist nurses, all supporting you and ensuring you are comfortable.

What to expect when someone is dying of cancer – the final days

For the individual who is dying and for the loved ones surrounding them, it is completely natural for both parties to feel a number of mixed emotions such as fear, worry, sadness, anger, panic or resentment. It may help you to talk to your family or friends, a healthcare professional from your team, a religious or spiritual figure or someone from a support centre.

There will be physical changes and emotional changes in the days and weeks before your loved one dies. These have been discussed in greater detail and Cancer Research UK provides invaluable information and sources of support for this difficult time (see Useful Resources).

9

Immunotherapy, targeted therapy and getting through treatment

We are living in an era of hope, as new cancer treatments, including immunotherapies (also known as biological therapies), are being developed all the time. Immunotherapy and targeted therapies are sometimes used to treat advanced or stage 4 CRC currently. They can be used as single agents or in combination with chemotherapy.

What is immunotherapy and targeted therapy and what is the difference?

Targeted therapy works by targeting specific parts of cancer cells, parts that help control the way cancer cells grow, divide or spread. Some targeted therapies will stop signals between cancer cells, stopping it growing, others will stop new blood vessels forming, meaning cancer cells can't spread (metastasise), and others will stop the hormones that allow a cancer to grow from connecting with the cancer cell.

Our immune system works to protect the body against infection, illness and disease. It can also protect us from the development of cancer. The immune system includes the lymph glands, spleen and white blood cells. Normally, it can spot and destroy faulty cells in the body, stopping cancer developing. However, a cancer might develop when:

- the immune system recognizes cancer cells but is not strong enough to kill the cancer cells
- the cancer cells produce signals that stop the immune system from attacking them
- the cancer cells hide or escape from the immune system.

Immunotherapy helps our own immune system target and kill cancer cells. Some immunotherapies are also targeted therapies.

Can I have immunotherapy or targeted therapy?

Eligibility for either depends on the type of cancer you have, the stage of your cancer and other treatments you may have tried. These therapies tend to work for individuals who have mutations in specific genes such BRAF, MMR (mismatch repair genes) or RAS.

Working out if you have a mutation and which one/ones allows a targeted treatment to be used can be done by looking for these markers in cancer tissue sample or sometimes in the blood to determine which type of immunotherapy would work against the cancer. Below are some gene mutations and treatments that may be appropriate.

RAS genes

RAS genes help cells grow, survive and multiply. If the cancer has a normal RAS gene, it is known as RAS wild type. If it has a mutation, it is called a mutated RAS gene. There are different types of RAS genes called KRAS and NRAS. You will need a blood test to see if you have mutations in both of these RAS genes. About 50% of people have some form of RAS mutation.

If you have the wild type RAS gene, you may be able to have the targeted treatments, cetuximab (Erbitux) or panitumumab (Vectibix). These treatments are not suitable for patients with mutated RAS genes. Both these drugs are EGFR inhibitors which means they stop cancer cells getting messages to stimulate them to grow. They are often given in combination with chemotherapy.

Side effects include: *allergic reaction (see below), skin reactions, diarrhoea, hair changes and sore eyes.

Mismatch repair genes

Some bowel cancers develop due to mutations in the genes that usually repair DNA. These are known as mismatch repair genes. These bowel cancers often have a high number of mutated genes. This is referred to as deficient mismatch repair (dMMR) or MSI-High (microsatellite instability). If you have this type of mutation, you might be able to have the immunotherapy drugs nivolumab (Opdivo) or pembrolizumab (Keytruda). Clinical trials are in progress looking at the

---

* Allergic reactions – more common with first dose (flu-like symptoms, drop in blood pressure, feeling sick).

development and role of other immunotherapy drugs in stage 4 bowel cancer, and at other stages which may avoid the need for surgery, chemo, or radiotherapy.

This drug blocks a protein called PD1 on certain immune cells called T cells, blocking PD1 signals to the T cells to find and kill cancer cells. It is used for those with advanced bowel cancer who have not had any treatment as yet, and have a high MSI or MMR deficiency.

BRAF genes

BRAF genes help cells grow and multiply. If the cancer has a normal BRAF gene it is known as BRAF wild type. If it has a mutation, it is called mutated BRAF. The most common mutation is called BRAF V600E. If you have the wild type RAS gene and the BRAF gene, you may be able to have cetuximab and panitumumab. If you have the mutated BRAF gene, the drugs cetuximab and panitumumab are unlikely to work. If you have the wild type RAS gene but a BRAF V600E mutation, you may be able to have the drugs cetuximab with encorafenib and/or binimetinib.

Side effects vary from person to person but can include flu-like symptoms, fatigue, skin rash, pain around the needle site, diarrhoea, vomiting, weight loss, rapid breathing.

Angiogenesis inhibitors

These drugs prevent cancer from developing a blood supply, hence starving it of oxygen and nutrients. Examples are:

Bevacizumab (Avastin)*

Aflibercept (Zaltrap)* (although available in Scotland)

Ramucirumab (Cyramza)

Regorafenib (Stivarga)*

Side effects: bleeding, blood clots, high blood pressure, small risk of bowel perforation, risk of infection, anaemia, chest pain, skin rashes, diarrhoea, constipation, poor wound healing and an underactive thyroid.

All the above drugs are given intravenously apart from Regorafenib which is taken as a tablet orally. Your oncologist will discuss whether they think you are suitable for any of them.

---

* Drugs that have not been approved by NICE in the UK so are not routinely available on the NHS.

If you have any problems with treatment, please let your specialist know.

Do speak to your oncologist or cancer nurse about your individual treatment as there are so many therapies becoming available and many that are currently being studied in trials. If you are not eligible for a particular treatment through the NHS, you may be eligible for one through a clinical trial.

This is a very scientific topic, and an intense part of our journey, and to put the treatment into context, Sophie has written about her experience of immunotherapy for advanced CRC.

Meet Sophie, diagnosed with stage 4 bowel cancer aged 36.

Sophie

Being diagnosed with stage 4 bowel cancer was awful, but it might have been what saved me. The first thing I needed was surgery to remove the tumour, and a biopsy of the tumour determined that I had the BRAF v600e mutation, and that I was MSI. The BRAF mutation causes a very aggressive bowel cancer, with the median survival rate being between 8–12 months, and it occurs in around 10 per cent of bowel cancers. Being MSI or dMMR (deficient mismatch repair) is uncommon, only occurring in around 5 per cent of bowel cancers, so to have both is not often heard of.

My oncologist started me on the strongest chemo (FOLFOXIRI) available and he also was constantly looking out for anything that might work for me in the background, even in clinical trials.

When my chemo failed, my oncologist referred me to the drug company BMS, which was looking for people like me, BRAF and MSI, to try a treatment that had been very successful in melanoma BRAF patients.

The drug company funded my treatment and I started a couple of months after chemo stopped. In that time my cancer had rapidly started growing again. It turns out that people who are dMMR or MSI are usually resistant to chemo, so it never had much hope of working for me.

I was moved to a new hospital and new oncologist. I was to have a dual immunotherapy as the cancer was so aggressive. Most people just have one immunotherapy drug. I started with nivolumab and ipilimumab for the first four cycles, which were every three weeks. After four cycles I moved to just Nivolumab, every two weeks from then on. As the treatment was still in the early stages (only a year into trials), they didn't really know what to expect for sure. I was told the treatment would probably be palliative. I was also warned that with having the two drugs, I had about a 40 per cent chance of getting any auto immune disease (normally it's around 20 per cent). The list of side effects was longer than the chemo one; some people had had skin problems, arthritis, colitis, vomiting, headaches, fatigue, and I could get some that were life threatening that would stop my treatment, but I was willing to risk anything to give this a go.

When I started immunotherapy, I was still suffering the side effects of chemo. I had lost a lot of weight, didn't have an appetite and was weak and fatigued still. I had nausea and fatigue for the first couple of days after immunotherapy and that was really about it. The time of my treatment had gone from 8 hours on the iv at the hospital and 48 hours pump at home to just 1 hour in the chair.

I continued the fortnightly dose of nivolumab with no further complications. My CEA (blood indicator for some) dropped down from 2900 at the start to 3, which is normal levels, and my scans were stable.

As I approached two years of treatment, I asked if I could have a PET scan as I had read of a couple of others having this done, and their tumours showing as dead tissue. The scan results were amazing. Absolutely nothing cancerous showing in my whole body. The next day I met with a liver surgeon who was willing to operate and get the dead tumours out. I was told that BRAF is so aggressive that I would never be able to have surgery as I couldn't be off treatment long enough.

Surgery was successful and I was deemed in remission by the surgeon. He couldn't believe how well the immunotherapy had worked.

Since then I have had PET and MRI scans every three months, as there have been occasions where the cancer has returned in some patients up to a year after stopping the immunotherapy. But fortunately for me that has not been the case and I have just passed a year of being in remission.

Immunotherapy is now available on the NHS as first line treatment for MSI patients, which is incredible. It has saved my life.

As I said at the beginning of this section, we have most definitely entered an era of hope.

Clinical trials and research

We are fortunate to live in a world where there is ever-evolving research into cancer, prevention, earlier detection and new treatment lines. With regard to treatment, there may be studies involving new drugs, new combinations of drugs, and trials examining side effects, cost effectiveness or comparing drugs used for symptom control.

You may be asked to take part in a trial, to help expand knowledge around cancer, but also to facilitate the development of new treatments, which may not be available to you otherwise. You will also be carefully monitored during and after the study. You also may be interested in participating in treatment trials and again, researching and talking to your specialist team to see what you might be eligible for is useful.

I was enrolled in two clinical research trials which were discussed before I went on to start treatment. The research team were incredibly friendly and knowledgeable and actually the doctor who was working as a research fellow at the time, and who was involved in both the studies, became a familiar face and a source of support through treatment.

It's important to have all the information to hand when considering entering a study, and to write down any questions or concerns you may have. If you decide not to take part in a trial, your treatment will not be affected; let staff know so they can address any concerns you may have.

You may also be asked to give permission for your blood sample or tumour sample to be sent off for research purposes. This research can take years but again can improve what we know about cancer and its treatment and hopefully alter the outcome for patients in the future.

Getting through treatment – day by day, step by step

'Believe you can and you're half way there.'

Theodore Roosevelt

You now know what treatment you will be started on, you have an idea of the side effects that may accompany it, and quite frankly you may be raring to get going. This section will hopefully give ideas on how to keep going through treatment cycles, when you might be struggling, feeling flat, ill or deflated.

Prepare yourself

General advice resembles that given earlier in the book. In addition, ensure you have enough stoma supplies and medications from your doctor and have the kit ready to manage any side effects.

Visiting a chemo suite if you haven't done previously is also a good idea. This gives you a chance to meet the team who will be administering treatment and hopefully it will demystify any concerns you may have. There are some people who are unwell on these units, but try to keep the focus that many more people undergoing treatment get better than those who don't.

Chemo units are extremely busy and, since the advent of COVID, there is a variety of restrictions in place so please check with your local unit if you are able to take a chemo buddy. I felt I needed the hand holding and took my brother or my husband. I was usually the youngest person on the ward and I felt a slight awkwardness till the nurses welcomed me. Some patients were keen to talk and share stories, others kept their heads down and continued with their business. I was given tips from long-timers on chemo, most importantly how to go to the toilet with a drip stand and chemo in tow!

Try to keep a routine – be a creature of comfort

This is not easy, especially on the days where you are willing every muscle to help you get out of the bed to the toilet, or you have your head wedged in a sick bowl. On the days I felt brighter, I would try to get up with the children, have breakfast and a shower, and rest a little once they were packed off to school. I would try to meet one person a day so I had some social connection and company as G would work long days.

I'd try to get some exercise, usually walking with a friend, but on my drug-free weeks, I would go to the gym or work out with a personal trainer friend, or go for lunch; I'd keep a list of Netflix programmes to watch, and try to rest or nap in the afternoon when the children returned home. Most nights, I was pooped and in bed by 7 p.m. Everyone is different but I found by pacing myself and sectioning the day into chunks, it was definitely more manageable.

The drug-free week – Hallelujah!!

If you do have a drug-free week in your treatment schedule, there are a couple of things to remember. This is the time to nurture yourself back to health as much as you can, so that you are fit and well enough for the next cycle. It is also the time to refuel mentally and physically as well as to eat well, and move!

Here is a journal entry from my first drug-free week.

December 2019 (cycle 1)
This week – well, between rest periods, I'm feeling better. I've been off my first cycle of chemo for six days now. I still usually need to go to bed around late afternoon but things are dramatically better than week 1. I still have migraines

daily – I'll speak to my oncologist on Friday about that. But generally better off the drugs! No surprise there!

On a positive note, the hand-foot syndrome (palmar-plantar erythrodysesthesia) quickly settled within 48 hours of stopping the capecitabine. Oh, the relief.

I was told diarrhoea would be more problematic on week 3 of the cycle from the capecitabine and it sure has been – Imodium to my rescue every time! Luckily, this symptom has not been as disabling (yet) as I first thought it would be. I was expecting armageddon, but I'm dealing with my normal of 13–14 times a day at best and at its worst 25 times a day. Sore bottom alert!

I've managed to get out and about, and I've managed to see a few friends which has been SO uplifting and importantly been to see my children's nativities in church yesterday. It certainly felt like Christmas and I'm totally embracing this week and the festivities till more chemo next Monday, which means I'll shut down for the week ahead on the run up to Christmas Day, with the incessant fatigue and side effects. I have some 'events' this weekend to see me through the next couple of weeks too and ensure I have my full dose of Christmas cheer and sparkle, and hope the tiredness and headache intermittently do not interfere too much with my agenda.

Refuelling – how to keep going on treatment

Trust me, there will be times when you want to give up and throw the towel in, times when you feel so awful, you feel utterly helpless. Refuelling on your 'week off' treatment is a crucial part of keeping going. This is also the time you can usually plan to fill up your empty cup, and get yourself ready, body and mind, as best you can for the next cycle of treatment.

It was just magic to see what a difference the following made to my wellbeing during these refuelling weeks (which will look different for everyone). I would try to plan activities each day, often simple and short-lived, so I could find time to rest and recharge, till the next cycle. Some of my highlights included:

- Friends turning up and taking me for a surprise – a change of scene
- A meal out
- Spending quality time, just the four of us, catching up
- Buying a new item of clothing or make-up – sparkly, of course
- Getting out of pyjamas and getting dressed up (more sparkles)
- Therapy/counselling
- A lot of giggles
- Time with the children, or family – quality time

- Nourishment – because while on chemo, my appetite was not good and I craved beige food
- A cheeky gin and tonic
- Getting out of my home town
- Escaping to the sea
- Playing my favourite sport or exercise, new walks.

It may have taken every ounce of energy some days to go out. However, one thing was consistent. I would go to sleep with a full and contented heart and a smile on my face. Feeling a piece of the old me. It would help me rebuild, and gain strength mentally, and remind me why I was doing this, and going through quite harsh treatment at times. This may sound peculiar, but there are times when one might feel so unwell, with moments of sheer desperation, there would be very fleeting thoughts of, 'Well, what's the point?' We all know the reason. Surrounded by friends, family or animals who love you for yourself, this is the reason to refuel. Ready for the next round. Ding ding.

Maintaining your identity

Cancer takes a lot away from you, including your identity. Some may argue appearance is superficial. But I think keeping up appearances and trying to look good, using make-up, clothes and so on, can be used as armour to combat cancer, which can take away your identity, self-worth and confidence, too. I made it clear from the start that I didn't want to look like I was unwell or undergoing any sort of cancer-related treatment.

1 December 2018
Cancer makes you feel vulnerable, and can negatively affect both your self-esteem and confidence. The scars, the illness, the mental fatigue, the drugs and their side effects, the way some people see or treat you differently. And the person staring back at me in the mirror isn't quite the person I expect to see these days. That person appears tired and drawn, somewhat lost, and has a constant air of bewilderment about them – that 'what the hell just happened?' look. They have thinner hair, fewer eyelashes and fainter eyebrows. Their skin is dry and imperfect too. The differences are subtle, but cumulative. And of all the medicines I take, I find these changes the hardest pill to swallow, because they signify a real loss of my identity.

Trying to look well on days I managed to get out of bed was so important to me. Even more so than before. In fact, I don't think I've ever bought so many sequins, trainers (dreaming of running again), and so much make-up (be it steroid-fuelled shopping in the early hours) in such a short period of time. Much of it was returned, to my husband's relief, bar sequins and sparkles!

But trying to put some glamour and normality back into my life was so important when, let's be honest, there were moments I could barely walk with tubes and lines hanging out. I'd be sitting on the loo for hours, not wanting to eat but only to throw up and sleep, hiding till the storm passed again.

And for my children, to see their mum, who used to like make-up and clothes, look like herself again was so important. I think they wanted to burn my baggy post-op comfortable clothes after I had my stoma reversed. And they did notice my change in appearance – 'When are you going to stop wearing pyjamas when you drop me to school?' Just to clarify, they were very, very nice jogging bottoms; nonetheless, this spurred me on further to try to take care of my appearance when I could.

This is not for everyone, however, and there is no obligation to dress up to the nines if that doesn't help you or make you feel any better. Finding your thing to maintain your identity, though, can help ease the process and make you feel like you have some control or ownership of your situation, whether that's taking care of your appearance, maintaining your exercise regime, looking after your garden, journalling or doing some voluntary work.

Taking care of your appearance in treatment (or finding your thing):

- can make you feel you have purpose
- can make you feel better about yourself
- can make you feel alive (even when you feel rough inside)
- can make you forget or hide the effects of cancer and its treatment effects, even if for a short while
- can make you feel more like you.

There are lots of websites around to help with this and ensure you choose products that are cancer friendly. I was fortunate enough to attend a 'Look Good, Feel Better' session at the hospital I was receiving treatment at, and I've shared my experience below. 'Look Good, Feel Better' is the only international cancer support charity that helps manage the visible effects of cancer treatments. Their website offers advice and support, and a range of 'cancer treatment'-friendly beauty products. They also offer a complimentary make-up and skin care workshop, as well as gifting patients with the most fabulous bag of products, which have been donated by a range of cosmetic and skin-care companies. Christmas had definitely come early for me, as I was fortunate enough to be offered an opportunity to attend a workshop through my cancer centre.

10 December 2018

In the session I attended, we had a brilliant hair stylist/make-up artist, who had the most fabulous sense of humour, as well as three other local beauticians. Each and every one of them a volunteer, donating their time, skills and expertise. They nurtured and supported eight cancer patients for 2 hours, and equipped them to 'look good and feel better' through their cancer journey.

I attended on a day when I felt dreadful. It was nearly a week after my first infusion. The nausea was overwhelming and I didn't think I would last the session. To be honest, I could just as easily have stayed in bed. But I'm SO glad I found my inner strength that day, because two hours later, I had eight new compadres with whom I had laughed and cried, as we piled on creams, potions and make-up, while sharing our stories. I couldn't actually apply a lot of the products, as my hands were so painful from the neuropathy, but the beauticians worked busily, performing their magic, giving us tips and advice about anything and everything, including how to best preserve facial features and skin through chemo treatment.

The lady next to me was in her 40s. She had endometrial (womb) cancer, and had suffered a stroke, so she found it difficult to communicate. She had lost her hair through cancer treatment and was wearing a head scarf. The therapist asked if she could remove it. She reluctantly agreed. But as it came off, she started crying, it was the first time she had felt safe to do this in public – such was the incredible power of this class. A total stranger to me, but I hugged her tight and shared her tears. She was far braver than me. I felt a fraud as I sat there, only a week into chemo, with my full head of hair.

I came out of the session feeling happier, more confident, less vulnerable, ready to take on the world with my full face of make-up on, armed with products, knowledge and ideas as to how to preserve 'me' in the coming weeks, and not to 'look like cancer'.

For any of you out there who have (or have friends who have) the big C, who may be struggling to maintain your identity, I cannot recommend one of these sessions enough and the unquantifiable difference to the lives of cancer patients.

Finally, before we end this chapter, this final piece looks at the bad days, with extracts from my journal that cover the times I really struggled. Please feel free to skip over this section if you might find it triggering or disheartening, and continue with the positive energy from the pages above.

Christmas Eve, 2018 – cycle 2

3 a.m. This week has been the absolute pits. I can't even begin to describe HOW ILL I feel. This is torturous, I can't stop crying. I can't sleep at night, I'm wired on steroids, yet in the day, I'm so lethargic and bed bound, willing every muscle to get me to the toilet. It's an effort to eat and drink. I know I've got to drink, as I stare at the pot of herbal tea thinking, I wish I could just have a drip with fluids right now.

I literally feel like I'm rising from the dead. And it's Christmas Eve and I'm determined to be Christmas ready for my children. So I find my big girl fun pants and get ready to throw myself into the day. The symptoms all seem to settle a little, the acute sensitivity to cold, the nausea and lack of appetite, the muscle pains and cramps, the fatigue, and generally just feeling atrocious. My mood lifts, having spent much of the previous few days in tears, wallowing in self-pity, paranoid ideas and anxiousness, feeling so so lonely – I wonder if it's partly due to the drugs or the fact I just feel so unwell, and that I can't socialize or sit out of bed for any length of time. As soon as I can, I try to function as a mother first and foremost. I start to eat better which helps with my general wellbeing and although I've gone off any meat during chemo, I manage a small amount of Christmas dinner, even though some flavours still make my taste buds curl up. I spend most of the afternoon languishing by the fire just soaking in all the joy of Christmas hoping that, for just one day, my family can forget about the reality we are currently living in.

We have a quiet but wonderful Christmas Day with my brothers and mum too and I manage to push through the day, just grateful that I'm sitting upright. I know I've overdone it, as I feel faint by mid-morning on Boxing Day and have to take myself off for the rest of the day. Either way, I'm so pleased the children and my family have had a lovely Christmas and soon I'll manage to walk further and start exercising once more.

15 January 2019, cycle 3 – a new low

It's been a while… I'm not having a good time right now. I've had relatives die of cancer-related illnesses this week, and people I know have endured new diagnoses of cancer. Cycle #3 has well and truly poisoned me. My mind too. Telling me to stay positive won't help right now. The drugs have dug their filthy claws into me. Making my mind weak. It transpires that I probably succumbed to my children's stomach bug/gastroenteritis, and the nausea and diarrhoea have been something else, so chemo has been stopped temporarily. And I'm on black alert to attend hospital if I spike a temperature.

This has been the hardest cycle so far. Maybe due to the cumulative effects of chemo, but also due to the infection I've been harbouring. I've been in bed for seven days straight. I'm so lonely, yet I don't want company. I feel like I can't go through much more of this. Yet I'm desperate to restart my chemo and finish this cycle.

133

And when my husband asks 'how do you feel?', I tell him I think I've caught a glimpse of what dying feels like. Dramatic as it may sound. But it's the only way I can describe it. And in a way, this is true. The chemo is killing me, cell by cell, the good ones and the bad ones.

So shit. Cancer.

This whole sorry story.

And the children, my husband, my beautiful family ... we are so solid, but the cracks are starting to show. And my motherly guilt is at an all-time high.

My petrol-warning light must be broken, because the tank is running on empty.

Can't afford to break down now.

Hope we get there soon. x

Be prepared for the bad days and know this day shall pass.

'The days that break you are the very days that make you.'

Unknown

PART 2
LIFE AFTER COLORECTAL CANCER

10

The aftermath – life after cancer

February 2019

There is light at the end of the tunnel and the end of treatment is in sight for sure. This comes with a bag of mixed emotions – of course I cannot wait to finish … no more surgery, chemo, possibly fewer side effects and less pain, but the five-year surveillance does begin and also the knowledge that 'it' could come back at any time.

I felt my heart sink momentarily when I was reviewed for the last cycle of treatment. My very brilliant and lovely oncologist said the next time I would see her would be in eight weeks to discuss my first CT scan result. Reality hit hard, with the realization that the comfort and bubble of my weekly to thrice weekly jaunts to hospital will be no longer, and I will have to integrate myself back into my 'new normal' life. The cancer specialist nurses are always there and will be my first port of call, but why I do feel as if I have been suddenly released back into the wild?

Which led us on to talk about life after cancer treatment, 'survivorship', and 'how do you move on from something like this … how do we want to live our life from here on in?' This is the million-dollar question that I'm still trying to work out, and will need a lot more time to cogitate over, once this last cycle is under my belt. For the last time, I hope, it's time.

Taking those last chemotherapy pills, my children cheered. I waited expectantly as I thought I should be feeling relief, a sense of achievement and the need to celebrate. And I did feel this momentarily, but I also felt stunned as I paused and wondered what on earth had just happened over the past seven months – the rug having being pulled, well and truly, from under my feet. I did indeed feel elated for the first few days following treatment ending, as the immediate effects of chemo started to wear off, and I did decide to celebrate, trying to ignore everything that had happened over the last few months. And, after enjoying the moment with my children, the first thing I did was throw a party with my dream team locally who had supported me and helped us day to day! It was a celebration and a huge thank you for helping us through the last few months. Of course, within this room full of happiness, there were lots of sparkles and sequins, I was dancing on my chemo-battered feet, rushing to the toilet several times, sending a friend out for emergency Imodium (rookie error) and taking a seat next to the dance floor when it all got too much. None the less, it was an incredible high – but what I'd learnt already was that there were often incredible lows that followed, and the brutal reality of finishing treatment would strike eventually. It will hit. And, when it does, it hits hard. That this part of the road trip is just the beginning of a new phase… the new normal, the 'life after cancer', the aftermath. Where there will be a need for more determination, grit, patience, perseverance. There will be tears, and joy. Taking all the small wins each day and through the bad days, remembering that tomorrow is always another day.

Survivorship

Contrary to what many may think, survivorship starts from the moment a patient is diagnosed with cancer. It encompasses anyone with a cancer diagnosis, whether treatment is ongoing, or the cancer has been cured, or there is an advanced cancer diagnosis.

A person who has had cancer is sometimes referred to as a cancer survivor, regardless of the course of their disease. Not all people like or use this term so it is important to acknowledge this according to individual preferences. Many stage 4 cancer patients refer to themselves as 'thrivers' – again, these terms are personal preferences.

Survivorship aims to focus on health and wellbeing, and includes assessing the physical, emotional, mental, social and financial effects of cancer on an individual, from diagnosis, through treatment and beyond. Every person affected has a unique experience. A key theme within survivorship is trying to regain aspects of your life before cancer, as well as finding and paving new pathways resulting in fulfilment and a satisfactory quality of life ahead.

Survivorship care plans can be documented and discussed with your health care professional.

The Useful Resources section has details for a survivorship care plan document that has been set out by the American Cancer Society and outlines the diagnosis, treatment received, side effects, long-term effects and follow-up. It also includes lifestyle advice and how to live well moving forwards.

In the UK, there is a Holistic Needs assessment which also encompasses some of these aspects. See the Macmillan website for further details (see Useful Resources).

I've finished treatment – what next?

Finishing treatment also signals the start of recovery. The time to try to get back to 'normal', whatever that may be. It's where you roll your sleeves up, and get ready to muck in. It's where the real work starts. Some may feel like celebrating. Others just stare disbelievingly into the abyss. It may feel 'done and dusted' to those around who jubilantly praise you and want to paint the town red marking the end of treatment. Everyone feels very different emotions and you may want to pause and allow yourself to feel whatever you are feeling – after all, you have just been on a treadmill, never really pressing the red 'Stop' button.

What can actually surface around this time is all the trauma, emotion and grief that have been building up since diagnosis and through treatment.

There are some people who appear to sail through life after cancer and integrate back into their normal, but this is the minority. For most, it is not so straightforward. It is important to take stock of where you are at and start thinking about where you want to be, what important aspects will contribute to your recovery, and to be kind to yourself, taking one day at a time, as you enter your 'new normal'.

A new normal

When it comes to a new normal, this simply acknowledges the changes in life that follow a crisis or traumatic event such as cancer, where life as you knew it before the event no longer exists in the same form.

Living a 'new normal' after a traumatic event such as a cancer diagnosis or treatment is the most frightening and tumultuous rollercoaster I've ever strapped myself into. Inevitably, it can be a confusing time and there is a lot to get your heart and head around. Many end up feeling lost, worried, abandoned and alone, during what is a confusing and uncertain time.

I had never fully appreciated that life as I knew it pre cancer would change forever. My goal during treatment had been to keep some semblance of 'normality' for the family and power through it as soon as I could, in the hope I could 'go back to normal'. In retrospect, I'm not sure how well I achieved this but that was probably more a reflection of my expectations I had at the time. Little did I know about this 'new normal' and that the Anisha post cancer had in fact been very changed. And that, now, I may just have to adjust my sails. This is a normal response to living through trauma and, later, post-traumatic growth would follow, an entity which helps build and reshape your new normal (see Chapter 18).

A new normal can encapsulate a variety of changes – as a person – physically, mentally and emotionally, but also your perspective, your thoughts, your feelings, your reactions, your empathy, your life goals, dreams and wishes. In fact, it may feel as if your whole life plan has been overturned by cancer. Do not fret, the old you won't be completely lost, and there will be a blend of the old and the new you to varying degrees, differing from person to person. I'd like to call ourselves 'upgraded'.

So, when it came to navigating a new normal, was it easy? No.

Did I like it? Not initially.

But do you have to find a way to go forth and make sense of it all? Yes, as well as living and hopefully thriving. And ultimately, there is a life after cancer and beyond. Maybe without rose-tinted glasses, but with gratitude-filled ones, instead!

For me, contemplating this new normal felt overwhelming, despite the fact I had survived cancer. I felt I had shed enough tears along the way during treatment, surely there couldn't be more? Truth be known, I've been through a whole host of emotions during this time. There have been periods of healing, self-care and therapy, fighting with times of self-sabotage, burnout and exhaustion. I've also been through the stages of grief for life before cancer many times over (denial, anger, sadness, guilt, despair, and now acceptance – most days).

The fact that I should be grateful I survived cancer, but found myself a mess post treatment, with a new perspective and a wealth of side effects physically and mentally, made some days very challenging. And so much had changed. Why did it have to change even more? Let's face it, not many people like change. We are, after all, creatures of comfort.

Despite what may feel like many obstacles, with setbacks along the way, it is possible to integrate back into society, mingle with friends and family within your new normal, return to work, possibly have a family (even if not by traditional routes), to find happiness and feel a wealth of gratitude once more. And personally, I think I've grown, and maybe even blossomed as a person because of cancer, as clichéd as it may sound. I think more positively about making the most of my new normal and every achievement is so much more precious and valued.

Milestones are more sacrosanct, and memories more cherished.

Much of what I write here comes from my experience and also from what I've learnt from others. What I do know is that how people are affected by their new normal falls on a spectrum, with some people not really being affected, to those who feel they have found a new calling and life. Most people are somewhere in between.

With a lack of information out there about life after cancer, it's so important to raise awareness of this and to share. Coming to terms with the fact that life after cancer is different from life before cancer is a monumental step in recovery.

For anyone struggling with their new normal right now, that's okay. It can be the absolute pits, it's isolating and it's lonely, and I see you. I hope this chapter highlights ways to start thinking about your recovery.

This is an extract I wrote three years after treatment ended, touching the tip of the iceberg of the 'Cancer Aftermath'.

The cancer aftermath ...
During and after cancer treatment.
> The fallout.
> The collateral damage.
> The aftermath.
> Is just too big for words.
> And I, as well as many others out there, still get floored by many of my symptoms some days.
> Some more common and collective – mental health wise.
> Something an Instagram photo often won't show.
> The invisible disability.

The reality of going to the toilet. More times than you can imagine. The pain. The urgency. The anxiety it can induce. The LARS (lower anterior resection syndrome, or bowel dysfunction post rectal/bowel surgery – see Chapter 12).

Managing when I eat at times, or when I run, many having to manage what they eat too.

The nagging pain from sciatica.

Burning in my feet or hands with cold.

The mental anguish with time has diminished but triggers unexpectedly letting the adrenaline rip through my veins driving me into fight or flight mode.

I often get asked, 'How do you work?' 'How do you manage symptoms?'

To be honest, we learn to live with this new normal.

We learn tricks to manage and cope. By endlessly trawling the net, therapy, asking friends, looking at support groups, trial and error because actually the help needed doesn't exist to the degree it should.

And three years on, all these things have improved to varying degrees. But all the above still haunt me at times. Sometimes one or the other … occasionally all at once.

Which pushes me to a tipping point.

Where the gratitude of being cancer free is sometimes difficult to palpate.

And the grief, anger and upset of the life BC that no longer exists overtakes.

The frequency of which, I'm pleased to say, has lessened.

What I personally always try to remember though is tomorrow is another day. I dust myself down, maybe have a wee cry, then put on my make-up, wear something bright, exercise, plan fun things, and try to dampen down the noise of cancer.

I've grieved the loss of my life before cancer, and now turn my hands to positive causes in the life I have been given back.

And I am genuinely grateful to be here.

Because that's all I can do,

To keep living this chance at life and embrace what I've been given.

Because it has opened my eyes, a new perspective with many new opportunities.

And for that I am truly thankful.

Life after cancer sometimes gets easier, and it sometimes bites again. Recovery is never linear, as we know. But, on the whole, having a box of tools and trying to find the rainbows, sparkles and gold dust in this new normal is how I, personally, find a way forward. On the days I can't, I know tomorrow will be another day, where hopefully I can.

My patients also never fail to inspire me. I had a wonderful chat with an elderly patient who had finished cancer treatment a couple of years previously. The consult we shared is vividly etched in my memory, because everything she told me she felt was so relatable. From feeling so lonely and like suddenly she'd been dropped from all hospital care, to feeling the last few months were just a surreal blur.

She was incredibly upbeat, admitting there were dark days too, but she had been given a second chance to 'get living' and was planning to take up a variety of activities that she had been meaning to do, as she recovered. Never mind being almost 90 years old! It was impressive but, having known her for years, I was not surprised by her tenacity and inspiring attitude.

'Why didn't anyone tell me it would be this hard after a cancer diagnosis and treatment?'

March 2019
No one told me it would be this hard after treatment finished.

No one. And there is no manual. No instructions when you're dropped from your swaddling blanket of hospital care. Comforter removed, pacifier thrown to the kerbside.

Things have changed for me now though.

Things are different.

I see things through different glasses. An altered perspective.

As I'm thankful to just be here alive and breathing.

When I fell off the treatment conveyor belt, there were thoughts of worry racing through my head. Concerns over:

- My mental state
- My physical state
- My ability to slip back into life – trying to rebuild a life after cancer. Do I try to pick up where I left off, or do I even want to do that?
- Addressing the issues and people that I have had to 'park' during chemo.
- My tolerance of people 'sweating the small stuff' and their 'first world problems'. That people will expect more of me than I can offer right now because I may look fine, albeit shattered, and have finished treatment, but inside I feel vulnerable, exhausted and broken.
- That the huge support network of both my medical and non-medical team (friends and family) will drift away.
- The five-year surveillance period we are entering.

I fully recognize I need time and space to reflect, to breathe and to recover both physically and mentally. And how long will this take? The million dollar question. Well, I just don't know.

So why is it so hard, after a cancer treatment?

Learning to live and cope with the long-term side effects of treatment and cancer.

The loss in muscle mass and exercise tolerance.

The life-zapping fatigue.

You've had a lot of time to think, life slowed down in many ways while on treatment, and actually you're not feeling like you want to get back on the hamster wheel.

The impact on mental health and the prolonged emotional burden.

The processing of cancer, treatment and what actually happened – let's be honest, there is a lot of baggage to process, check in and then send on its way. This takes time and space.

The uncertainty and fear for the future, and your own mortality, has been brought to the forefront of your mind. The fact anything can happen to anyone at any given time.

The cancer admin can seem relentless and ongoing.

Falling off the conveyor belt from hospital follow-up and active treatment.

Self-identity issues – loss of identity, low self-confidence, low self-esteem, who am I in this 'new normal'? I felt I had lost my identity as a doctor, a wife and a mother and these were all the things I felt I needed back to feel 'normal' and complete.

Grief for your life before cancer.

Worries financially, about employment, housing, and social issues

Strains on relationships, revaluation of relationships.

A change in your life plan – your expectations, of how life may pan out, your goals, your aspirations, for some everything they feel is mapped out. Cancer drops a bomb from a height on this, and causes chaos, and one may feel forced down another route temporarily, till the smoke has cleared and you can reassess what your life plan may be.

A NEW PERSPECTIVE. I found this really challenging. On the one hand, I was so pleased with the gift of these 'new glasses'. A new lens. A different outlook on the world around me. Things looked more Technicolor, I was certainly more grateful and I knew I never wanted to sweat the small stuff, I wanted to embrace life with both arms and do EVERYTHING! I would say to myself morbidly, 'I'll sleep when I'm dead!' However, the flip side to this were feelings around people who to me didn't appear to value life the way I did. I would become frustrated with people worrying about minutiae, including my loved ones. How could they possibly be fussed about the colour of their curtains? There is obviously nothing wrong with wanting the perfect curtains, but clearly this was a reflection on where I was at that moment of my life and what I had been through. I couldn't make sense of such trivia having faced something so vast and I didn't like feeling this way, and I didn't like myself for feeling this way either.

How to begin to recover after cancer

No matter how you feel when treatment ends, it is time to breathe and to process, and to think about recovery. Broadly speaking, recovery will involve supporting your physical, mental, emotional and social wellbeing.

This is also a time where sometimes you can need just as much support as you did during treatment, yet it's a time where this safety net can fall by the wayside. The majority of those affected by cancer find treatment easier than the path after treatment for a number of reasons, many of which I've listed above.

How do you cope with this new normal and life after cancer?

'Adopt the pace of nature, her secret is patience and knowing that spring always follows winter and the sun follows the rain always.'

Ralph Waldo Emerson

There will be good days and bad days.

Set yourself small, achievable tasks or goals each day. This builds your confidence, rather than setting unrealistic goals, which may knock your confidence or make you feel like you've failed. Try setting yourself a short walk each day and build up gradually. Or set a goal to eat healthily. And remember, don't compare yourself to others.

- Give yourself time to get to know the new, upgraded you.
- Be honest with yourself and others about the way you are feeling, what your new normal may mean in terms of your ability to go out, go back to work and so on.

- Kick the guilt to the kerb. As we'll see later, it is a wasted emotion.
- Focus on the here and now.
- Set realistic expectations.

Tips: Coping with life after cancer

- **Pace your activity:** I know I was so eager to get back to normal, do everything for my children, meet up with friends, start exercising, and think about work all at once. Don't feel you need to take on everything simultaneously. Increase your activity one step at a time, listen to your body, take the naps you need and don't plan too much in the early days. Don't be afraid to still ask for help.
- **Eat well, exercise and sleep:** Many people diagnosed with cancer become more health aware than before. I have noticed a flurry of people who became vegan, vegetarian, stopped buying certain products to help obtain some control potentially over the future. Ask your doctor and research trusted sources to understand how to reduce your risk of recurrence. If you know you are living a balanced, healthy lifestyle, know you are doing all you can to reduce your risk.
- **Focus on your own wellbeing and self-care:** Be kind to yourself, this is a huge undertaking, and do not underestimate it like I did. Put your own life jacket on before you help others. Healing starts with you, and then with your immediate loved ones. It was a very unusual situation to be in, and one that was mentally quite tough – putting myself first, instead of being the wife, mum or family doctor. We will talk more about this.
- **Reassess life priorities:** This is a good time to decide what your priorities are, how you would like to move forward… a less stressful life? Different job? Healthier lifestyle? Take up new skills you've been talking about doing for years and just never got round to?
- **Rest guilt-free:** Listen to your body. If you need to sit down and rest, do so.
- **Access services or specialists:** This means those that you think may help you rehab or manage the 'new normal'. For example, I tried acupuncture for my sciatica and peripheral neuropathy, I had counselling to manage the psychological aspects post cancer, I had physio to help rebuild my strength and for the sciatica. In some ways I think having this 'therapy' offers a crutch from when you are 'dropped' by the hospital post treatment.
- **Be honest with those around you…** and don't forget to reach out and ask for help if you are struggling.
- **Talk to your doctor:** Always ask your doctor if you need any support, or help with the management of side effects.

- **Lean on your team:** Your team is your community, your army – tap into your abilities and gather all the tools you can to help you rebuild.
- **Keep coming back to this chapter:** It may be that you're not ready to fully embrace the new normal as you need time and space to process, but revisit it when you're ready.

Finally, and most importantly, recovery is not linear. Figure 9.1 represents expectations of my energy levels and progression (as well as regression) as I reached various milestones.

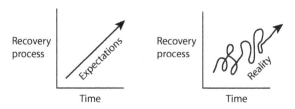

Figure 9.1

'Just be' – the cancer noise

There is an inherent noise from cancer which is amplified a million times to a deafening level during treatment. When treatment ends, you hope the volume will be turned down.

When I did finish treatment, however, no matter what I did to distract myself, the cancer noise was still booming in my ears, and this vexed me. I felt I had served my time during treatment and I just wanted to get going with life, to live life; what I hadn't appreciated, even as a doctor, were the battle wounds that ran deep, mentally and physically. I couldn't be objective, I couldn't use my 'doctor head', I don't think I'd even started to process what had just happened.

So, I tried to let it be. My husband would find me at home or whenever I was by myself in a room with the music on full volume, with never any time for peace and quiet. I love music, but this behaviour became an obsession, one that my husband couldn't initially understand – until I explained to him that I didn't like being alone, or alone with my thoughts, and the loud music drowned out all the cancer thoughts in my head.

I started to research and invest in things that would potentially aid my recovery. Acupuncture and vitamin B6 high dose for my peripheral neuropathy from chemo and sciatica, physiotherapy for my sciatica, Pilates to strengthen, and regular counselling to try to make sense of all these emotions, which I just didn't have a handle on.

As the acute chemotherapy effects started to wear off, I jumped back on the bandwagon of everyday life, in an unrestricted way. Before I knew it, I was exercising, reconnecting with friends, trying to eat well again, and taking naps, all the time dealing with 'cancer admin' and appointments. I struggled with not having a normal routine and life, my impatience always getting the better of me as I watched the world go by as if nothing had happened. The problem stemmed from the fact that how I wanted and needed to portray myself back in the real world did not tally with how I felt inside. Which led to me feeling misunderstood, many people thinking, 'oh she's fine' when I wasn't. There was a lot of unpacking and processing that needed to be done.

I learnt to master the mute button over time, and cancer was – and still is at times – packed away in a box, only to come out for special occasions, such as the loss of someone I know who had cancer, or certain triggers, scans or follow-ups. Of course, in my day-to-day work, blogging and even writing this book, it is at the forefront of my mind, but only occasionally does it turn up the bass of emotions like it used to previously.

Forward planning

When can you start planning? Whenever you feel it is right for you.

I used to find this extremely unsettling in the early days after treatment. Not only was cancer and its treatment a full-time job, the aftermath was, too, and it really is a job like no other. One that would leave me feeling pooped by the end of the day, cancelling plans last minute. I felt I would never be able to plan anything again, and we lived between surveillance scans. As time goes on, the focus has changed. The scans are still there, but the cancer noises do become quieter as the days pass. You settle into a routine that works for you, maybe return to work, go on holidays and return to the hobbies and sports you love. And slowly, I have found myself starting to make plans, without second guessing the 'what if?'.

Following on from this, I thought it might be useful, here, for me to share some of my journal entries over time, looking at the progress during this time and highlighting the fact that recovery is not linear, but that time, tools and space help not only with healing, but also with moving forwards. These are clearly snapshots of moments in time and obviously doesn't represent how I felt day in day out.

Three weeks after treatment ended

Going back to hospital almost filled me with a perverse joy. It felt comforting. It felt safe. I thought this was slightly odd, but the counsellor reassured me that many patients feel this way after treatment.

I'm just a flat tyre with too many punctures right now. The 'aftermath' certainly perplexes me. I fear the post-chemo tiredness, and how long it will linger. I'm not really sure what I'm meant to feel. Partly I think it's the chemo fatigue. Too tired to think about anything else. But my son has also been having a tough time this week. He is confused, angry and sad and it's almost as if he has had an epiphany about what we have all been through and is grieving for us all. It has been heartbreaking to witness and it's all come out this week. So, I spoke at length to my counsellor about all of this and we are doing our best to help him through this.

We also discussed the fact I've completed seven months of very intense treatment with little time for recovery between each stage.

And I never had a second to breathe, time to ponder, to recover physically or mentally.

I've been told by fellow cancer patients, my counsellor and oncologist that often when treatment finishes, the reality of what you have been through really hits you. Bang! Crash! Game over. You're done. And I've seen this all too often in patients I have cared for in the past too. I'm still waiting for this moment.

So now, I'm filled with anticipation as I fall off the conveyor belt back into the world that once ran me ragged.

I'm under no illusion, this bloody cancer has hit me hard, both mentally and physically. The promise of the 'old Anisha' returning when treatment ceases may remain unfulfilled. I'd love to see her again in her Technicolor glory, but some days, the signal being broadcast seems more black and white. The physical insults will no doubt take time to recover; the psychological ones, longer still.

What I do know is that I need to spare a few seconds in my AC life. Time to take in the ambiance and enjoy the view. Life should be full, but not uncomfortably so.

A valuable life lesson.

I'm just fearful of the future, so am nervous to make any plans.

Too busy juggling with unknown variables.

And trying to work out how to recover and find my way.

But my heart is totally there with everything. We need the plans and 'events' to keep looking forwards, to live life to the full, to continue making joyous and beautiful memories.

Six weeks after treatment ended

You would have thought a clear scan, a couple of fabulous holidays and my portacath removal today would be enough. I should be over the moon. These were highs and yes, I am.

But this cancer malarkey just keeps on giving in many other ways that others can't see. The physical scars may have healed but this week has seen the start of my crash downhill. The long-awaited downturn. Back to reality. You think you have nailed it and are moving forwards but it infiltrates, working its way in like a parasite and the emotions come flooding back. Jeez.

Many people may take an emotional dip around eight weeks post treatment – I'm six weeks post treatment … I always like to be first! And seemingly this is probably what's happening. And I know I need to be patient, kind to myself and give myself time, but I am the most impatient patient.

I prematurely stopped counselling for the last six weeks as I thought 'I was fine', drifting in my bubble of 'fine'. But I've started it again this week and for the first time, I cried through my whole session. Grieving for normality. The loss of control over our future and what we have been through is bringing consequences. I've been keeping myself ridiculously busy and wearing myself out to try to avoid thoughts. Obsessing over a healthy lifestyle to regain some control in my life. My mind is a discord of anxiety-filled thoughts vs insights with rational solutions. Constant battles in my head.

I can't go an hour in the day without thinking about cancer.

I don't feel I can plan more than six months in advance.

I feel like keeping my portacath in 'just in case' I might need it again.

And all this is because I think it's finally sunk in. What has happened. Grieving for my old pre-cancer life and not knowing how to move forwards. Or to make sense of it all.

I know I have many positive opportunities out there now that I can grab. And all to live for. With the billion thoughts in my head, I am desperately just trying to gain some clarity. And I know this is just another blip and all part of the process. I know I just need TIME.

Three months after treatment ended

I'm still trying to piece my life together. Cancer, you really did turn it upside down. … and despite me trying to do damage control as much as possible, it's going to take time. I just feel like I want a break from it all.

Sometimes people just don't understand, even those that are close to you.

This was my biggest fear post treatment and one that as time goes on is becoming more prominent.

They don't understand why you suddenly feel sad, when you were laughing two minutes ago. They don't understand why you are still tired (often quite abruptly to the point you have to stop your activity immediately). They don't understand why you take pictures all the time (ensuring memories are captured). Or why you have the music turned up loud (to avoid your own thoughts).

Someone gave me a great piece of advice …'If you are on a plane and it's about to crash, put your oxygen mask on first, before you help your loved ones and others.' And quite frankly I do feel like we have been in a plane crash.

As The Greatest Showman said, I wish I could rewrite the stars, but from now on life is like walking on a tightrope, so I make no apologies at all, because 'THIS IS ME'.

One year after treatment ended

11 February 2020

It's been a tricky and painful few days. Stormy. Much like storm Ciara. Entered a dark hole of flashbacks and trauma going back into hospital for the spinal injections for my crippling sciatica and then a LOT of pain since, spending most of the past few days in bed. That loss of control I have being a patient and not a doctor still gets me every time. This is also what happens when I can't keep busy. Argh. Those thoughts coming back again where I'm scared about the future … be it pain that never goes, or cancer again. Usually tucked deeply away in my brain. Too much time to think. I can't even take lots of painkillers because they upset my bowel.

So I turned to the water and dragged my arse to my swim club today in the hope that water usually relieves the pain temporarily. And it did, to a degree, as well as filling my cup and lifting my spirits. It's just as well as I have an important talk tomorrow!

12 February 2020

This time last year marked my last day of chemo. I had a lot to be grateful for. Today I went back to where I trained as a GP. I stood up and told my story, your stories, to a room full of strangers, listened to stories from others, and imparted medical education. Feeling even more gratitude as this has injected me with three things:

1. Clarity that this is exactly what I want to do. Raising awareness with the platform I have with health professionals, seeing the difference I can potentially make. There are times I have questioned whether this is good for me. I got my answer today. Yes. It is. Yes, there is heartache that comes with it at times and writing this talk was emotion-evoking – but I know if even one GP listens to one thing I've said today and it changes patient care/decision making – it is totally worth it.
2. Calmness – for being able to talk openly about me, my story, my future. About the emotional and physical rollercoaster. It was a release that I so needed. But I managed to hold myself together the whole way through, my voice only wavering momentarily a couple of times.
3. Confidence – that I CAN do this. I can't even begin to say how amazing and liberating it was to stand up today in a room full of doctors/trainees and talk for two and a half hours straight through an interactive talk with future GPs about cancer in the young. Telling my story, telling the stories of others from the grid, sharing experiences that I have learnt from you

all, the pitfalls, the trials and tribulations. How we can learn from the cases I shared. Spreading awareness about CRC in the young. Talking about screening (focusing on bowel and cervical today) and ensuring they understood what it involves, its limitations and its challenges. And where we can help in primary care. How we can do better. For our patients. To ensure earlier detection, diagnosis and vigilance through doctor education but also public health promotion. And how we can balance all this with time, pressure and resources in the system we work in. And I think they learnt a lot. I'm feeling really high at the moment, natural endorphins as painkillers – some days, I feel like I'm static, but today is reminding me just how far I have come.

The COVID pandemic struck one year after I had finished treatment. I had returned from the holiday of a lifetime to South Africa, a belated 40th birthday trip, and I was feeling rejuvenated. However, on returning to the pandemic, I very much felt this changed my course of recovery. Initially, it gave me purpose, almost swopping one C for another and, as a frontline worker, I felt all my energy channelled into crisis mode, rather than focusing on cancer. I also had more time to exercise in the initial months, as there were fewer commitments – apart from work and home schooling – and my physical and mental recovery was no doubt aided at times by this.

However, I started to burn out, as did many others. Work was presenting a continual stream of triggers, and so there was no better time to embark on a course of trauma-based CBT.

18 months after treatment ended
September 2020
Today I finished a 13-session course of trauma-based CBT. I have tears of joy because I turned up, and persevered, because those who know me well know I've struggled with it at times. The therapy initially caused my mood to dip completely into a deep, dark hole. However, I'm pretty sure it's made a difference in both my professional and personal lives and I'm doing so much better.
    Mentally
    and
    Physically.
    I was very fortunate to have a fantastic relationship with my NHS therapist and she congratulated me today on my engagement and determination to see this through, during a difficult time. Another hurdle overcome after cancer and I feel really proud. I'm not suddenly fixed and I can still feel teary thinking about cancer, but the blow has certainly been softened. As the therapist said, we will never be able to take all the pain away, but I've certainly been empowered with

tools to deal with my new normal and many different triggers. The ultimate test is the coming month, with it being follow-up and scan time once again.

It was fantastic to see my PTSD score come down from 39 at the beginning of treatment to 17 at the end.

And at its highest, my anxiety scored 15, which seemed to peak after reliving certain experiences (it got worse with therapy before it got better), but today the score was 3.

So it got me thinking to this time last year and where I am now. The list I reeled off to my therapist, reminding me that I'm one of the lucky ones:

My fatigue is less

My fitness has massively improved (in fact I've just managed my first half marathon up Leith Hill!)

My neuropathy continues to improve

My sciatica is improving/more manageable

My anxiety and panic are less

My resilience has increased

My confidence and self-worth have improved

My emotional lability and tearfulness has lessened

My LARS is improving/more manageable because I know the triggers for me specifically and how to use medications to control this if needed. Like all of us who suffer, we all get caught out now and then still.

And importantly, I'm starting to look to the future (cautiously).

I think we have fully established that life after cancer is complex. In this latter half of the book, we'll look at ways to help with the process of finding a new normal in all the rubble around you post cancer, as well as supporting your physical and mental wellbeing during the aftermath.

11

Exercise and fatigue – how to get going

Exercise, or physical activity, should most definitely be a modality of cancer treatment, high up there with chemotherapy, radiotherapy, immunotherapy/targeted therapy and surgery. From the moment you are diagnosed, through treatment and beyond, ensuring you participate in physical activity is key. Every minute of movement or exercise counts, with a huge number of benefits attached.

Prehabilitation

What is prehabilitation? It is the process of improving the body's capacity to undergo cancer treatment through a programme of help and support.

From the minute you hear the words 'You have cancer', it is important for you to consider your physical activity. It may be the last thing you feel like doing but being more active and exercising is a major part of prehabilitation. This is a programme of advice and support that can help to prepare you for upcoming treatment. The other parts of prehab include eating a varied diet, stopping smoking and looking after your mental wellbeing. Your doctor can signpost you to help with any of these areas of concern.

Cancer treatments are often compared to running a marathon; in the same way it's advisable to train before running a marathon, it's important to increase your physical activity before you have surgery, radiotherapy or chemotherapy.

We do also know that if you spend some time focusing on exercise, your mental health and diet, prior to treatment, this can:

- give you back some control
- help you manage better during treatment
- promote a quicker and better recovery.

As well as all the other, longer-term benefits of exercise, by making it part of life with cancer, it can help you to live well in the long term.

Research has shown that you can build muscle mass, strength and fitness in as little as two weeks, so don't be put off by thoughts like 'What's the use? I've not got long till treatment starts.'

I fully appreciate this may be totally overwhelming at a time of complete shock and upset so be realistic and be kind to yourself in terms of what you can achieve. If you are ever concerned about exercising at any point during and after cancer, please do discuss this with your healthcare professional.

What exercise or physical activity should I do?

Everyone has different starting points, so set realistic goals for yourself. Remember there are people that have been at the same starting point as you and they have been able to manage. You can do this. And remind yourself that being physically active means any movement that uses your muscles or more energy than you would when you are sitting still. Therefore, it can be as simple as taking the stairs instead of the lift, dancing, gardening, or walking. Not everyone has to march themselves off to the gym or go out running!

Where possible, it is more beneficial if you can aim to exercise as outlined below.

Current advice recommends 150 minutes of moderate-intensity activity or 75 minutes of vigorous-intensity activity every week, but my advice is do what you can, and on the days you can't, it's ok, don't beat yourself up.

Note: Moderate-intensity activity results in you feeling warmer and breathing faster, but still retaining the ability to talk. Activities include brisk walking, cycling, gardening or housework. Vigorous-intensity activities will cause an increase in heart rate and you will start to sweat and feel out of breath. For example, running, aerobics and fast cycling or other types of exercise.

Tips: Physical activity

- Once cleared to do so by your surgeon, return to normal daily activities as quickly as possible after surgery.
- Build up slowly, in terms of time and intensity.
- Listen to your body.

- Resistance or weight training twice a week – building muscle is important before your cancer treatment. Muscle mass is also linked with your diet. With regard to this, it is important to try to get enough protein in your diet as well, at least 70 g a day.
- Remember to incorporate stretching.
- Remember to work your core and pelvic floor especially if you've had pelvic/abdominal surgery – I highly recommend pilates post-op. It provides strength training, fitness, flexibility, aids balance, reduces pain as well as strengthening your core and pelvic floor at the same time, which is so important in bowel cancer patients.
- Incorporate yoga or balance exercises into daily routine. Some chemotherapies causing nerve damage can also affect balance! I noticed this, and even catching a tennis ball when I first started playing after treatment was really tricky, as well as any balance exercises! Yoga is also good for relaxation and stress management.
- Try short, frequent bursts of exercise, at a time of day that works for you.
- Enjoy.

What can I do if I am finding being active difficult?

Remember to be clear with yourself that physical activity is a type of therapy for cancer. Imagine it as a pill that you've been given on prescription. Plan your activity through the week at a time which is best and most convenient for you. Have a timetable.

Keep a diary of your physical activity – so you can keep track of what you are doing and congratulate yourself on your achievements. It also allows you to think about ways of being more active if you aren't quite getting enough in.

Exercise with someone (not for everyone), but this can give you accountability and help ensure you turn up, while keeping it fun, social and connecting at the same time.

Think about what is keeping you from becoming or staying physically active. For example, you might feel tired, you may be feeling depressed or suffer with a lack of confidence or motivation. Decipher ways to overcome the barriers you're facing, or get the help you need. Join a class to stay motivated. Think about exercising at a time of day when you're less fatigued.

Choose an activity that you will enjoy and that is local to you. I initially became self-conscious, especially after surgery, so chose to exercise at home and take regular breaks. I remained a member of the gym and would choose off-peak times. I also took my physio with me to give me an exercise programme that built my strength and muscle mass and a friend who was a personal trainer regularly helped me train.

I took the plunge and joined a swimming club with others of all abilities to spruce up my swimming technique and help with my sciatica, while placing the running on hold. It was a real confidence boost and I met an array of individuals including others rehabilitating after cancer.

I also asked friends to come and get active with me. Activity with others provides social connection, motivation and camaraderie too, which is most definitely therapy in itself.

Exercise after surgery

Trying to restore my core muscles post major abdominal surgery, stoma formation and reversal was hard, hard work. Many thought I was premature revisiting the gym but I took what exercise I could on the 'good days', first and foremost to keep me sane.

Unfortunately, after treatment ended, I completely overdid it. I'll admit this now. Having had months of little exercise that I was previously accustomed to doing, having had major abdominal surgery twice and then cell-killing chemo, I very quickly got straight back into high-impact exercise ignoring what treatment had inflicted upon me physically, not fully realizing the deconditioned state my poor body was in. At the time it was my way of coping. But the excessive nature of the exercise I undertook resulted in a number of injuries, and a recurrence of the sciatica that I had at diagnosis, with recurrent ankle injuries not helped by the fact I am hypermobile. On top of that, the exhaustion that would ensue … I would exercise in the morning and feel great, nap in the afternoon and then be asleep by 7 p.m. each day. I didn't know when to stop exercising, and just kept pushing. Why? Because it made me feel alive and forget what I had been through. And that the 'old' me was still there. Strong. Fit. Active.

The stoma nurses helped immediately with exercise programmes for the first six weeks but after that, I trawled the internet to little avail and went off piste doing my own thing. Maybe I would have avoided injury and been in a better place had I had more information, both mentally and physically. But getting the right balance and not pushing too hard is key.

So, on a wise person's advice, I binned my fitness watch in the hope that I would listen more to my body than I did to a device. Subsequently, I worked diligently training four times a week to regain my strength and muscle mass, recondition, improve my core and glute (buttock) strength to help my sciatica. Most of this was under rehab programmes specifically targeted to my weaknesses by NHS and private physiotherapists. We made videos and I watched my progression over the months, slowly increasing weights, the complexity of exercises and working on endurance. I would remark to my physio that I found it really tricky to feel the right side of my core where my stoma had been, I felt it was difficult to 'fire up' or engage, probably as a result of the nerves severed during surgery. Despite this my sciatica worsened and I was plagued with pain, unable to sit down for any length of time. I was referred on to a pain clinic eventually and given injections of steroids into my spine, almost like an epidural. I had to try something as we were due to fly to South Africa for a delayed 40th birthday trip and there was no way I could even sit for 30 minutes, let alone a long flight. I'd also been given the news that I would probably never run long distance again and would find it difficult to ride a bike or spin with the state of my sciatica, and it may sound petulant, but I mourned the loss of activities I loved doing with family and friends. Swimming and reformer Pilates filled the void along with strenuous workouts on the cables, cross trainer and the BOSU, my new bestie. The BOSU exercises look easier than they are – but really activate the smaller muscles in our body that aren't often exercised, and I would highly recommend.

There are so many people out there who can't do the exercise they want to for a variety of reasons, but what's important is you tailor a regime that works for you and your body.

You never know how your body will respond and recover with time. Low and behold I did get back to running and lockdown gave me the time to get fitter and fitter and stronger and stronger and, as we came out of lockdown in March 2021, I undertook my first half marathon up Leith Hill, and in October that year, my first London Marathon, and it felt tremendous. A real milestone. Never say never.

Exercising through chemotherapy

I tried to exercise as much as I could through treatment. Spinning, resistance band workouts, slow short runs, long walks, TRX machines with the help of some incredible people who kept me going, motivated me and adapted exercises to my treatment phases.

Staying active after diagnosis and through treatment (when it allows) is so important. Don't get me wrong, there were days when I didn't get out of bed. And I just could not fathom moving. But when I could, I clutched the opportunity with both hands and literally ran with it. Because I caught glimpses of the me before cancer. And because I know there are plenty of health benefits from exercise during treatment too. For example:

- mood – reduces anxiety, depression, improves self-esteem and empowerment
- improves general physical functioning
- reduces fatigue and can result in increased energy levels
- reduces pain
- reduces risk of cancer recurrence (breast, bowel, womb)
- reduces risk of heart disease, diabetes and so on
- improves quality of life
- prevents or improves lymphoedema
- develops better bladder and bowel control.

Depending on cancer types and treatments, some people might need to avoid certain types of exercise or take extra care. Always ask a health professional if unsure.

Exercise is definitely a modality of cancer treatment. And once you get back to exercise in whatever shape or form, I wholeheartedly believe you will never take exercising for granted again.

Cancer-related fatigue (CRF)

December 2018

The fatigue I experienced was like no other. The plug had been pulled out at the mains and the lights had gone out. I found the fatigue itself psychologically injurious, and damaging at times. I missed the gym, running, pilates, bootcamps, swimming and just frankly having enough energy to sit up with the children or friends and family. I missed my sense of achievement, although some days, frankly just 'existing' and making it through to nightfall seemed to be the biggest achievement of all.

However, walking and yoga and resistance training seemed to be the way forward to combat chemo-induced fatigue. A friend started some resistance training to help preserve my ever dwindling muscle mass. My disappointment, that I could only lift a fraction of the weight I had been able to prior to surgery, was a blow. What did I expect, seriously? It's bad enough when you miss exercise for a week, but having been through all this, my weakness was evident for me.

I continuously hoped my muscle memory would kick in, in the knowledge that keeping active through chemo on the better days would help me in the long run, as well as with the fatigue. It felt so good to be back in Lycra, accessorized with gloves and hiking socks of course, to ward off the cold-induced nerve pains. I'm not quite ready for 'the plank' yet as my abdominal wounds are still healing, and my core is shot from the surgeries, but no doubt I'll be on it again soon.

I've already noticed a positive difference in my mindset and fatigue levels, so for now, I'll power on through with the walks (once my feet are better for the hand and foot syndrome from capecitabine chemo) and continue resistance training when I can, and accept that I need to batten down the hatches in week 1 of my next cycle, ready to fight another day in week 2. At the back of my mind, I know the side effects of chemo and the tiredness from all I have been through are cumulative … but for now …

I will try to focus on the here and now …

Till the next cycle.

This was a passage from my journalling after my first cycle of chemotherapy. I knew I would be fatigued but had no idea how floored I would feel and how the activities of one particular hour or day could impact the next so significantly. What I will say is that everyone experiences this to different levels and if you feel incredibly fatigued, this is not a sign of failure, as there are so many variables that contribute to the fatigue and response to treatment.

Fatigue in cancer is multifactorial and the list below highlights contributing factors:

- Post-operative fatigue: pain, healing from a major operation
- Treatment-related fatigue: chemotherapy, radiotherapy, immunotherapy, targeted therapy

- Insomnia: secondary to drugs such as steroids, and secondary to stress and the mental health impact of cancer, toilet trips, stoma changes, pain, side effects such as vomiting
- Reduction in fitness and muscle mass
- Appetite reduction or dehydration (I remember the days when even getting a glass of water used just too much energy)
- Emotional stress and poor mental health
- Anaemia – low red blood cells (haemoglobin) responsible for carrying oxygen round your body.

Fatigue after chemotherapy tends to occur soon after treatment and the days following, improving by the end of the cycle. With each cycle, the fatigue levels did increase and it took longer to shift, but the treatment-free week really provided an opportunity to refuel and get active!

We know that patients who expect to feel fatigued are more likely to, so wait and see how you are during treatment and don't second guess how you might feel.

Tips: Managing fatigue

Managing fatigue is very much a multi-pronged approach:

- Work out what worsens and what can improve fatigue.
- Pace activity.
- Ensure there are no medical causes of the fatigue such as low blood count, pain control if in pain.
- Address any mental health issues.
- Eat a balanced diet.
- Sleep well – see the Appendix for more on sleep hygiene.
- Take daily exercise.
- Prioritize, plan and pace – see below.
- Self-care.

Boom and bust

April 2019 – the rollercoaster

The struggle continues between the highs and the incessant need to live life and get back to it versus the consequences of being burnt out, often leading to complete exhaustion and ongoing emotional turmoil. This is very much the 'boom and bust cycle' and can really affect my emotional wellbeing in everyday non-cancer life as well.

> The slightest thing could overwhelm me when I get to the 'bust' phase. Some of my friends are starting to notice that actually, I'm not fine, that tough exterior that I try to maintain as a way of coping has been hard to maintain these last couple of weeks. I'm not ok.
>
> It's just too much, some days, and all I want to do is disembark this roller-coaster, but it's just not that easy.

'Boom and bust' is a concept where you might feel like you're on fire, undertaking activities galore (the 'boom' element), fluctuating with episodes of under activity and absolute exhaustion (the 'bust' element). It can also apply to pain and fatigue.

I threw myself into activities, but was also mindful of needing rest. When my body stopped, it just came to a grinding halt and I would find myself collapsed in a heap. With time I tried to tune in and listen to my body moaning in exhaustion.

Many people throw themselves into high levels of activity when they feel good, which can lead to setback, exhaustion and several days of inactivity while recovering.

So, what is the key? Pacing. Pacing allows you to take a balanced, consistent and steady approach to activity to, hopefully, stop swinging from one extreme to another. Over time, activity can then be increased.

Principles of pacing

Prioritize

Does it need doing today?

Does it need to be done at all?

Could someone else help to do it?

I'll talk about self-care shortly but this is essentially about prioritizing your energy reserves for the activities that are really important, be it work, a wedding, a hospital appointment, your child's school fete. I had to actively think about what my priorities were for each day, say 'no' to things – which was a novelty – and ask for help when I needed it. Self-preservation is key.

Plan

What do I need to do to carry out the task?

What time of day is best to carry out this task for me? When am I at my best?

What does the task involve? Concentration? Walking? Listening? Sitting?

When on active treatment, it is worthwhile bearing in mind when fatigue will be worse, for example, at the beginning of each cycle, and as treatment progresses. Fatigue can also continue for several months after treatment has ended, but there should be a definite improvement two to three months after treatment.

Pace

Can the task be broken down into several stages that can be done over time?

Taking the above into consideration, I would hope that having this structure to work from could help you to plan your days and weeks to try to avoid the bust days as much as possible.

Self-care

This is a term that is becoming increasingly popular, and I for one am so pleased that this is the case. Having a title for guilt-free time to do something kind and caring for yourself physically, mentally and emotionally is never more important than after a cancer diagnosis. In an ideal world, this should be an effortless part of living.

Looking after your own wellbeing is the priority before you can think about looking after your family, going back to work, and so on. Always secure your own life jacket before securing those of others.

Have a think about what self-care looks like to you. Make a list of things that ease your mind, relax you, something that is just 'for you'.

Here is my self-care list:

- Exercise
- Mindfulness – in the form of cooking, swimming and tennis!
- Sleep
- Walking in nature
- Pilates or yoga
- Reading a book
- Getting my nails done/having a face mask
- Spending time doing my hair or make-up
- Journalling/gratitude journalling
- Asking for help if there is too much going on

- Dancing like no one's watching
- Saying 'no'

Think about what self-care looks like. Other suggestions include:

- Gardening
- Social media break (digital detox)
- Trying a new hobby
- Doing a brain dump
- Listening to music
- Going on a date night
- Going to your favourite place
- Watching the sunrise
- Reading a book
- Listening to a motivational podcast or TED Talk
- Having a candlelit bath
- Buying yourself a bunch of flowers
- Call someone you love
- Go and get a coffee
- Book a trip away
- Have a bath
- Do something to make you laugh

We know self-care can help you manage stress, increase energy levels, reduce anxiety, protect your mental health, improve relationships and self-esteem as well as reducing illness and improving your physical wellbeing. What's not to love about self-care?

Sleep

Sleep is pivotal for healing and convalescence mentally and physically. Being chronically deprived of sleep can impact mental health negatively and can lead to anxiety and depression, as well as increase the risk of physical illnesses such as heart disease, diabetes and high blood pressure.

What people often don't realize is that how we behave from the moment we get up can impact how we sleep that night. From the amount of exercise you take, sunshine you see, medications you take, and the food and drink that is consumed, as well as the bedtime routine, all of these can impact sleep.

In the Appendix, you'll find more on sleep hygiene, giving you tips and self-help to aid better quality sleep.

Growth mindset

'A pessimist sees the difficulty in every opportunity; the optimist sees the opportunity in every difficulty.'

'Success is not final; failure is not fatal: it is the courage to continue that counts.'

Winston Churchill

With all the above, it is important that we harbour a growth mindset way of thinking rather than being rigid or fixed in our thoughts. This means we try to shift our way of thinking from seeing a problem as an obstacle to seeing it as an opportunity, to potentially make change, for example.

Someone with a fixed mindset may say, 'I'm so tired, I've been through so much, I can't exercise.' Someone with a growth mindset will say, 'Right, this is tricky, I'm feeling so, so tired, how can I help myself, who can I ask for help? Although this is tough right now, let's try to overcome it.'

The language is strikingly different and with a growth mindset, you are more likely to implement positive change, grow as an individual, learn from your experience (good or bad) and do better long term. It turns what is perceived as failure on its head so instead, we develop, grow and learn from the experience.

Even when the dark days came, and I felt ready to surrender, in the back of my mind, I would constantly be thinking, what can I try next cycle to make things better? Who can I ask for help? How do I get my fix of exercise? How do I feel less isolated? Problem-solving rather than feeling drawn in by the problem itself. I feel my growth mindset has developed further due to my experience with cancer.

Tips: Achieving a growth mindset

- Firstly, you need to want to make the change from a fixed to a growth mindset, having an open mind and attitude.
- Take risks and embrace opportunity – the fear of failure can stop you in your tracks when you see challenges as just this –

challenges, rather than opportunities. Be prepared that you will make mistakes, and don't be afraid to ask for help.
- Change your terminology – you did not fail at the task but instead you are 'learning' from the task.
- Allow yourself time to grow, learn from mistakes, and then grow again – take it at your pace and do not compete with others.
- Enjoy seeing others around you grow and flourish.
- Enjoy the process rather than just holding out for the goal.
- Keep persevering, practising and reflecting, your hard work will eventually pay off.
- And finally, remember the brain is malleable, so if the brain can change and adapt, surely we can, too.

And remember, there is always room to grow.

12

Lower anterior resection syndrome (LARS)

What is LARS?

LARS is a group of symptoms that occur after surgery for rectal cancer or reversal of an ileostomy, where either a part or the whole of the rectum has been removed. These symptoms can have a significant impact on quality of life after surgery, even when the cancer has been successfully treated. All patients who undergo bowel surgery will provide consent, prior to the operation, to accepting potential complications arising from surgery, including bowel dysfunction. I remember not even giving these complications a second thought when signing the consent form prior to my operation.

I just wanted rid of the cancer.

And now, not a day goes by when I'm not reminded that I've had rectal surgery. I'm not talking about the physical scars (I have very few of these as I had laparoscopic surgery). I'm talking about bowel dysfunction. A complete change from my usual bowel habit (which for me previously was once a day). And I'm well aware I'm not the only one struggling to manage these symptoms.

My head tells me it's ok – because it's not cancer. But my bottom says otherwise! There have been days where I've worried whether I will ever leave home and see the outside world again.

For some, it can have a real impact, to the point that symptoms are almost as bad, if not worse, as the symptoms of cancer itself.

The good news is that for most, the general trend is an improvement as time elapses from the date of treatment. Most will experience an altered bowel habit which can last for several weeks and take up to a year to settle down (sometimes longer) to a 'new normal'. For some, the symptoms may persist.

As I write, I feel I have got a reasonable handle on managing my bowel dysfunction most days, but in the early days, it didn't take much to upset the balance – the wrong food, a hot drink, alcohol,

or being abroad, illness, running … Regaining bowel con-
___ ...ving with a new normal bowel function is one of the biggest
challenges one will face after bowel surgery.

Why does it happen, and what can we do to manage this condition?

Why does it happen? The simple fact is that a segment of colon or rectum has been removed, anatomy has been disturbed, and nerve supply that co-ordinates bowel movements has been severed. And bowel control is a complex process.

The capacity of your rectum (the amount of poo it can hold) is less than it was before, and there is a reduced capacity for water to be absorbed back into the body. As a consequence of surgery, there is often poorer co-ordination of the muscles which help defecation, and an alteration in the function of the anal sphincter. It is possible there may have been direct surgical trauma to the anal sphincter during surgery too. And, without a shadow of a doubt, there is a heightened anxiety around 'normal' bowel function which serves to further fuel symptoms.

In most cases, time is all that is required for the anatomy to heal, the 'new' bowel to accommodate, and an acceptance of what constitutes 'normal' to allow a return to activities.

Patients are at an increased risk of developing LARS if the surgical join (anastomosis) was low in the rectum, if radiotherapy was administered, if an ileostomy was present for more than 12 weeks, in those over 75 years of age, and in those who had pre-existing bowel symptoms or disease.

For me, the awareness of my new bowel function became painfully apparent following my stoma reversal. It hit me hard. With my medic's hat on, I scoured the internet for hours, searching for information on the new evil in my life, seeking ways to tame it. And through my bowel cancer awareness work, I have had the pleasure of speaking to a plethora of colorectal surgeons, hoping that one may have the magic answer to my LARS, offering me a quick fix … But most are only able to admit that more research is required with regard to this post-operative beast.

Perhaps surprisingly, given its consequences, there is relatively little in the way of aftercare either available for or offered to patients with LARS. Underlying this is a paucity of research into, or controlled trial data regarding, the management of LARS. I was fortunate to be enrolled in a study investigating LARS and its impact on my quality of life when I underwent treatment at my local hospital, which required me to complete questionnaires on my symptoms and to score a quality of life rating. Hopefully, the tide is changing.

The colorectal specialist nurses are pillars of unwavering support in LARS. Ultimately, though, a strategy which works for one patient is often very individual to that particular patient, and an approach which one finds beneficial may not help another. Finding a way forward is often a case of trial and error – one size does simply not fit all. Our bowel habits are unique, and the impact of surgery varies widely between individuals.

Up to 80 per cent of patients with LARS report one or more of the symptoms below:

- Fragmentation (stools passed in 'bits') and a change in shape of the stool
- Urgency
- Incontinence
- A sensation of incomplete bowel emptying
- Frequency
- Tenesmus – a sensation of needing to pass stool, despite the bowel being empty
- Clustering of bowel movements (multiple bowel movements in a short space of time)
- Rectal pain – an inflamed or irritated sensation like a "hot rod" up my bottom
- Increased wind.

As you can see, the irony of LARS is that it manifests the very symptoms that took you to see your doctor in the first place!

From surveys of patients who have experienced LARS, 50 per cent report symptoms 10 years after surgery, and up to 90 per cent feel their symptoms have an impact on their long-term quality of life. From affecting your ability to work, to travel, to exercise, to going out, and even with an impact on sex drive and fear that a partner may have lost interest due to LARS – the effects can be significant.

At times, I've felt pretty alone with my symptoms, not knowing what to try next, or who to turn to for advice (and that's with my own personal gastroenterologist at home to bounce ideas off), and believe me, I've tried all sorts! So don't feel disheartened if you can't work it out some days either.

In my quest to find out more, I have found the following sources of information which may help fellow sufferers:

- Bowel Cancer UK
- A Facebook group called 'living with LARS'

How did LARS affect me in the year after my surgery?

This is me, one Friday in August 2019. Embarking on my night out. Here are just some of the thoughts trapped inside my head.

- Will I be late ... again? As I need to go to the toilet, AGAIN! (Get ready earlier)
- Where is the nearest toilet? (Google Maps)
- What if there is a queue? (I would take a 'need the toilet urgently' card out – see below)
- What if I'm on public transport? (Plan short journeys or stops!)
- If I need it urgently ... will I make it? (Take Imodium before leaving)
- If I eat out, will I get more symptoms? (Avoid things proven to aggravate symptoms)
- Have I got my meds? (Check, check, and check again! I keep a stash in my handbag, work bag and so on)

Addressing these head-on, and pre-empting the solutions (in the brackets above), gave me the confidence to go out with my shiny new cancer-free bowel and hope that it would all would work out.

Before we look at the management of LARS, there are a couple of conditions you should be aware of that can affect the bowel after treatment. Unfortunately there is a lack of gastroenterology specialists who specifically deal with the gut-related side effects of cancer treatment in the UK, even though these problems have the same incidence as a condition such as inflammatory bowel disease, for which most hospitals have one or two dedicated specialists.

Bile acid malabsorption (BAM)

This is a condition causing an altered bowel function, which usually manifests with urgent, chronic diarrhoea. Bile acids (which are normally stored in the gallbladder) are released into the small bowel following a meal and facilitate the digestion of dietary fats and oils. But a number of conditions – including cancer treatment (surgery, chemotherapy, radiotherapy) – can cause these to be poorly absorbed by the small intestine and they instead pass into the colon where they are an irritant to the gut. This causes diarrhoea which may be pale, greasy and hard to flush away and can result in variable colour stools (orange or green). Some people experience symptoms that can mimic irritable bowel syndrome, like stomach cramps or excessive wind and bloating.

Please speak to your doctor if you are struggling. They can organize a test called a SeHCAT test which can diagnose this condition, and dietary advice and medication, such as cholestyramine or colesevelam, may be prescribed.

Small intestinal bacterial overgrowth (SIBO)

I experienced this condition after treatment ended, and it took a while to get to the bottom of it, but fortunately for me, I had a gastroenterologist at home who considered this diagnosis and helped me obtain the right treatment for it.

Both chemotherapy and surgery can adversely affect the size and type of bacterial populations that live in our guts (SIBO), which can result in unpleasant side effects.

Symptoms include pale or foul-smelling stools, diarrhoea, tummy pains, bloating, reflux, nausea, heartburn and excessive belching and flatulence. Treatment of this condition usually comprises a short course of antibiotics, but probiotics can be used successfully too.

How did my symptoms present, and what did I do to help with the LARS?

I suffered (and still do to varying degrees) all the symptoms listed above. In the early days I used Imodium (loperamide). Frequently! Each dose would usually buy me four to six hours of relative peace before things kicked off again. I admit that it took me some time to feel comfortable taking drugs to control my bowels, because the side effects of my chemotherapy had rendered me so psychologically averse to taking tablets. Initially, I simply put up with my urgency and diarrhoea. But there were many occasions when my symptoms were relentless, causing me to miss family time and deadlines. And, eventually, I relented.

Four years on, Imodium is still my best friend, and we go everywhere together, even though I now seldom need to take it. I've also identified certain foods that I know may trigger LARS symptoms, but most of the time, I choose to eat everything in moderation, and I eat as much fibre a day as I can. As mentioned, the daily recommendation for everyone is 30g, and this dose has been shown to reduce the risk of bowel cancer. It's not easy to ingest this amount, especially when you have had bowel surgery, but challenging your bowel to small incremental increases in the amount of fibre is one way of avoiding Armageddon!

Here are some further tips I've collated from the resources available to help manage LARS. Do remember, though, as we've seen, everyone is individual, and a lot of managing symptoms is a process of trial and error.

Anal sphincter muscle retraining/pelvic floor exercises

I'll never forget my surgeon asking me about childbirth pre-operatively. I was initially confused. The significance hadn't clicked, until I understood why he was interested in my pelvic floor, and any tears or injury to the anal sphincter I may have encountered during childbirth.

It is so vitally important to strengthen these muscles (which are used for bowel control), thus preventing the leakage of poo or wind from your anus, either involuntarily or arising through profound urgency. Pelvic floor muscles also contribute to bladder control and sexual function. The bottom line (no pun intended) is that pelvic floor exercises do help, and their importance is not to be underestimated. They should be performed multiple times a day (the NHS 'Squeezy' app is a very useful tool). I suggest patients stick Post-It notes around the house to remind themselves, or do them while undertaking daily activities, such as washing-up or brushing their teeth. A continence nurse or specialist colorectal nurse can also assist you with these.

Specific exercises aiming at strengthening the anal sphincter are listed below.

Strengthening exercises

Sit, stand or lie with your knees slightly apart. Squeeze and pull up the back passage/anal sphincter muscle as tightly as you can, as if you are trying to stop yourself from passing wind. Hold tightened for as long as you can. Then relax for 10 seconds. Do not hold your breath or clench your buttocks or legs.

Repeat at least five times.

Endurance exercise

Imagine your anal sphincter as a lift/elevator. When the sphincter is squeezed tightly, it's reaching the fourth floor. When relaxed, it is resting on the first floor. Try to squeeze gently to the second floor so you can hold the squeeze for longer, rather than clinging on tightly to the fourth floor. Time how long you can hold this for. Then relax for 10 seconds.

Repeat at least five times.

Co-ordination exercise

In quick succession, squeeze your anal sphincter as tightly as you can, let go, do it again! Count how many times you can do this before you get tired, and aim for at least five quick pull-ups.

Try to perform these a few times a day, and as the muscle gets stronger you will find that you can squeeze tighter, hold for longer and do more quick pull-ups before you get tired.

Positive gains from these exercises will only become apparent after several months, and only if performed regularly, several times a day. As with pelvic floor exercises, remember to make them part of your routine, for example, when you're waiting at traffic lights, or brushing your teeth or seeing the Post-It notes.

If you are doing the exercises well, nobody will know what you are doing, so once you are confident doing them you can do them anywhere.

Diet

Tips: Managing dietary changes

Keep a food diary and identify triggers, noting down how your bowel responds to that food: do you develop wind, bloating, diarrhoea, anything else? After excluding any offending foods, try slowly re-introducing them back into your diet, just one at a time, in small quantities, to see if they produce the same effects.

Give it a day or two. If your symptoms do not recur, consider either increasing the amount, or adding in a small portion of another offending item, and assess the effects.

If diarrhoea is a predominant symptom – try to avoid fizzy drinks, alcohol, artificial sweeteners, and sorbitol-containing sweets and drinks (often the sugar-free options) and avoid deep fried foods.

If constipation is an issue, try increasing the amount of insoluble fibre in your diet, but do so slowly. If you develop stomach cramps, wind, tummy pains and diarrhoea, then reduce your insoluble fibre intake. In some cases, soluble fibres may be more helpful in tackling constipation, reducing bloating and wind.

For flatulence problems, avoid gas-forming foods (beans, cabbage, fried food). Try peppermint tea or cardamom seed. Chew your food slowly and thoroughly, which reduces the amount of air inadvertently swallowed during eating, reducing wind.

Eating smaller portions more frequently helps minimize symptoms for some, but for others taking large meals less frequently is helpful – only through a process of trial and error will you find what works best for you.

Different foods and their effects

Foods that stimulate the gut	Foods that can cause wind	Foods that help with loose stools or diarrhoea
vegetables: sprouts, broccoli, cabbage, cauliflower, cucumber, onions, radishes, spinach and sweetcorn	beans and pulses	apple/pear puree
bran and foods high in insoluble fibre	sorbitol/chewing gum	bananas
pulses and beans	vegetables	potatoes
popcorn and nuts	bran	white bread/pasta/rice
high-fibre foods	nuts	chicken and fish
alcohol – especially beer, wine, Prosecco	dairy and eggs	
sugar-free foods with mannitol, sorbitol or xylitol	beer and fizzy drinks	
spices		
energy drinks chocolate		

Hydration

Drink plenty of water. Aim for at least eight glasses of non-caffeinated fluid a day – this helps to avoid constipation.

Medications

• Loperamide (Imodium) – 2 mg loperamide capsules – adjust the dose until soft formed stool (Bristol stool scale type 4) and take 30 minutes prior to meals. For those who find even a 2 mg capsule too potent, liquid Imodium may be more easily titrated in smaller doses (like me) to individual needs.
• Fybogel/low-residue foods/psyllium husk (Metamucil) supplements – these bulk your stools and may reduce stool frequency.
• Peppermint capsules – can be useful in combatting flatulence.

Probiotics

Probiotics do not have an evidence base for use in LARS, but I have found them hugely helpful in improving symptoms of troublesome bloating, flatulence, and poorly formed and frequent stools. I found they reduced symptoms of clustering, too. I obtained a high-dose preparation from a local pharmacy, rather than those obtained in the supermarket. I also used them between rounds of bowel-toxic chemotherapy. I used VSL3, but there are others such as SYMPROVE out there too.

Counselling

Invaluable in helping deal with the impact of what life has thrown at you. Peer group support is also available; as I mentioned earlier, a Facebook page – 'Living with LARS' – may be helpful.

Reduce stress

It is so important to try to reduce stress. Minimizing stress can positively impact your bowel symptoms as well as your general health. We know that stress affects the bowel via the gut–brain axis. Exposure to stress impacts colonic motor activity (the speed at which the bowel works), which can alter gut microbiota profiles (including lower numbers of potentially beneficial Lactobacillus, all of which can culminate in the development of unwanted symptoms.

Ways to deal with stress may include mindfulness, taking long walks, yoga, meditation, and participating in exercise or hobbies.

Acupuncture

Some patients have found acupuncture helpful.

Bowel retraining

Generally reserved for those with severe symptoms that have not responded to other treatments. Your colorectal clinical nurse specialist may have information about this.

Alcohol

No doubt about it, and apologies, but alcohol worsens LARS symptoms. Fizzy alcoholic drinks seem to be the worst offenders.

Good toileting habits

Why aren't we taught this at school? We should all be taught this. Quite simply, we should be given instructions on how to poo properly!
  Guidance should include:

- Sitting on the toilet with your feet 20–30 cm off the floor on a stool, which helps to fully relax the pelvic floor and muscles around the anus, thus emptying the bowel more completely
- Sitting and placing your elbows on your knees and leaning forward
- Only going to the toilet when you need to go
- Listening to the urge (but know, with LARS, when to try to resist it to build up control)
- Avoiding constipation
- Not spending longer than 10–15 minutes on the toilet at any one time.

It can sometimes be difficult to differentiate between needing to pass wind or pass stool (even for those without LARS!). Sometimes, there are false alarms, and a heightened sensitivity of the bowel after surgery is thought to contribute to this. Over time, you will become more familiar with your bowel function and more confident about how long you can safely resist the urge. I remember my husband encouraging me to hold on to the stool a little longer each time the urge came, by using distraction techniques, and encouraging me to relax – easier said than done, some days!

Be prepared

The thought of going out with LARS can be daunting, and frankly overwhelming at times, so planning ahead and being prepared for all eventualities can help improve confidence and allow you to relax and enjoy your time out.

My suggestions include carrying a small changing bag (which includes a spare pair of underwear, toilet tissue and sanitizer) and a supply of Imodium, and gaining in-depth knowledge about the local toileting facilities (how many/how clean/how well-stocked ...).

Don't forget, you are also able to use disabled toilets if needed, and your Radar key or 'I need the toilet urgently card', see Chapter 7.

Skin care

Going to the toilet too frequently, persistent diarrhoea and anal leakage can all cause soreness around the skin of the anus. The sensation is very distressing. If you can remember what it felt like down there the morning after a hot curry, and then magnify that sensation by about a hundred, you will be on your way to understanding the levels of unpleasantness I'm referring to.

Protecting the skin around the anal canal is imperative. Use a bidet (if you have one!), use water wipes or extra soft tissue paper, wash around the anus with warm water, pat the area dry after washing as rubbing the skin will make the sore skin worse, and finally (if needed) use zinc and castor oil or vaseline as a barrier. Try not to use any other products, especially fragranced soaps or antiseptics, and avoid talcum powder.

Referral to a specialist bowel control clinic

If you're still struggling with bowel function and control after the above, please do let your colorectal cancer nurse or your surgical team know so that they can support you further.

Here are some brief descriptions of what may be offered, none of which I have any personal experience of.

Irrigation

Rectal irrigation is being increasingly used to manage LARS and patients who have used it find it extremely effective. It helps reduce physical rectal discomfort, constipation and leakage or incontinence issues by effectively emptying out the lower part of the colon. This allows some people to better manage their symptoms and to function more effectively at work, during social engagements, and with travel.

There are various types of irrigation systems available, but in essence warm water is introduced through a catheter placed into the rectum whilst sitting on the toilet. This warm water both stimulates the bowel to empty and physically helps to flush out stool.

Percutaneous tibial nerve stimulation (PTNS) or sacral nerve stimulation (SNS)

Bowel function is regulated by a group of nerves at the base of the spine called the sacral plexus. In theory, stimulating these nerves through gentle electrical impulses can cause an improvement in bowel symptoms.

Biofeedback therapy (BFT)

Particularly useful for constipation and stool incontinence. This therapy aims at retraining your bowel and anal sphincter muscles. The method provides patients with information about the activity of the pelvic floor muscles by way of a visual display. BFT is considered to be a safe and non-invasive procedure.

Seek help – you're not alone

After reading this, you may be feeling anxious about bowel dysfunction after surgery, but please, please remember that you don't have to suffer in silence. Although your bowel function may never return to quite what it was pre-surgery, it is so important to persevere with treatments. Remember that one size does not fit all, and above all, be patient. Although things are unlikely to improve significantly in the very short term, you can perhaps seek solace in the fact that the vast majority of patients do experience some natural improvement in symptoms over the first year after surgery as the body accommodates to its new anatomy.

13

Menopause and fertility

As I sat through a consultation with Dr Stewart, my oncologist, discussing impending chemo, she began to reel off a series of side effects. I gave an acknowledging nod to each one. She proceeded to ask us if our family was complete. I paused. We didn't want any more children but this question highlighted the extent of the havoc treatment could play. I looked at my husband and we replied that our family was, thankfully, complete, with little time to ponder the enormity of this question. The added caveat at the end of the side effect discussion was that I may end up in an early menopause, too. With my specialist interest in women's health, I immediately planned that, in this eventuality, I would be heading straight for HRT.

For many, though, this is not an acceptable side effect and is a huge weight to bear, especially for anyone diagnosed young, those who have yet to have a family, or not even thought about family, or for those who are not in a relationship. Compounding this, the prospect of losing the protection of one's natural hormones and entering menopause can be overwhelming. I have had insight into the lives of many patients who have entered this stage, and it is by no means easy for many without cancer, let alone secondary to a cancer diagnosis. I myself, while writing this book, have recently started hormone replacement therapy (HRT) for what again I feel is early perimenopause, due to treatment and I have had to process the fact that I am entering this stage earlier than many of my friends of my age, and experiencing many symptoms earlier than I may have done otherwise. Looking back, I think I've been suffering for some time but certainly I have felt an improvement in my symptoms since starting it.

It is often, unfortunately, the least spoken about side effect, as the focus remains on treatment. However, it is important to discuss fertility preservation methods with a specialist if you find yourself in a position of wanting children in the future, and it is important to be aware of the symptoms of menopause so in the eventuality of any symptoms, you can seek help from your family doctor or another clinician skilled in this.

Here we meet Olivia who tells us her story of navigating infertility as a result of treatment and early menopause.

Olivia (@oliviasgotguts)

I was diagnosed with stage 3 bowel cancer at 29 years old.

After my diagnosis, I was told I would need 25 sessions of radiotherapy sandwiched with six rounds of chemotherapy. Luckily for me, I had ten days prior to treatment starting to try to harvest my eggs. It had never occurred to me that the treatment that would save my life would also mean that my body could never create my own little human being. I came to terms with having cancer very quickly. But not carrying a baby? I found – and still find – that very hard to come to terms with. I never imagined I'd be thrown into a medically induced menopause at 29!

I had an ovarian transposition* before radiotherapy started to try to prevent my ovaries from being zapped. This was risky and I was told that they couldn't guarantee it would stop me from going into menopause. I wanted to give it a go, as I had heard early menopause wasn't fun. Unfortunately, eight months after my treatment finished, I found that I was going through menopause. It happened pretty much overnight which I found very hard to deal with. It started with hot flushes, I had to carry a fan with me everywhere I went and would wake throughout the night with night sweats. This led to many more symptoms including lack of concentration, lack of libido, vaginal dryness, difficulty sleeping and anxiety. Just what you want at 29 and newly married! I contacted the surgeon who had done my ovarian transposition and she confirmed that it was menopause. I was offered HRT and I was happy to go down that route if it helped with the symptoms. It took me a while to find an HRT that suited me. Even on the best HRT I have found for me, I am still not like I was before. And I miss that old me. But I understand how lucky I am to be here, so I am grateful for that.

After treatment finished, my husband and I had four frozen embryos and we were so excited to know that being parents was a possibility. However, we couldn't do the next bit on our own … we indeed needed a miracle. We needed a surrogate. This is when my incredible cousin came out of nowhere and gave us everything we ever wanted. She gave us hope. She offered to carry our embryo. The surrogacy journey included counselling sessions, doctor's appointments and treatment for my cousin. One week after the transfer, we couldn't quite believe our luck when we received a video from my cousin of a positive pregnancy test. It had worked. Our little embryo wanted to stick around and make us a mummy and daddy! In July 2020, two years after I had

---

* Ovarian transposition is a procedure which detaches the ovaries and fallopian tubes from the womb and places them into the abdomen away from the site where radiation will be applied, thus trying to prevent damage to ovaries, which in turn would affect fertility and induce menopause.

finished treatment, our little miracle, Monica, was born. Both my cousin and Monica are well and continue to have a special relationship and bond. I can't wait to tell her how special her Auntie is and the incredible way that she came to be Monica.

Menopause

Let's clear up a couple of definitions.

Perimenopause occurs due to declining levels of oestrogen (and testosterone) in the body, which can precede the onset of menopause. Symptoms can occur in this phase and periods will still occur although their pattern, heaviness and duration may change.

Menopause occurs when the ovaries stop producing oestrogen. It is when a woman stops having her periods (for more than one year if over 50, and more than two years if not). Natural menopause occurs around the age of 50. Both these phases can be precipitated by surgical procedures such as a hysterectomy, or treatments including chemotherapy and radiotherapy. But menopause is not just about hot flushes and mood swings. In fact, there are 34 recognized symptoms of menopause (at least) and, after treatment, any concoction of these symptoms could indicate that you could be perimenopausal or menopausal – but help is available.

Early menopause is where periods stop permanently before the age of 45, resulting in infertility.

Premature menopause or primary ovarian failure (POI) is a condition diagnosed in those under 40. The condition results in the ovaries ceasing to work as they should so the oestrogen levels dip and vary. The individual may still have irregular periods and there is a small chance of individuals becoming pregnant.

Blood tests can be requested to aid diagnosis of early menopause and POI.

We know that menopause has a colossal impact on many aspects of life which, in turn, can lead to a demise in quality of life, placing stress and strain on the following:

- Sex life
- Relationships
- Self-esteem
- Ability to work

- Ability to exercise
- Ability to sleep
- Mental health and mood
- Long-term health.

Figure 12.1 shows the symptoms that could be an indication of a peri-menopausal/menopausal state.

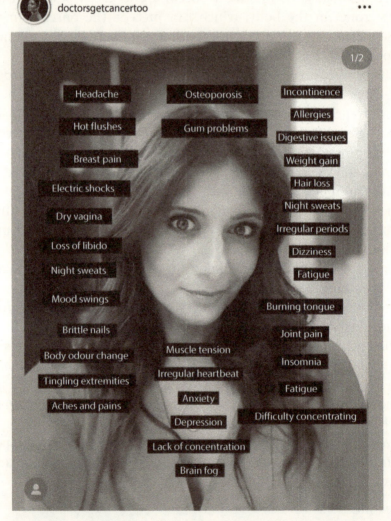

Figure 12.1 Indicators of menopause and perimenopause

*Osteoporosis is a reduction in bone density or thinning of the bones as a result of the drop in oestrogen. Osteoporosis can lead to bones fracturing easily if a fall is sustained.

It is always so important to seek advice from your GP because these symptoms CAN be managed and no one needs to experience them in addition to the aftermath of cancer, treatment and its side effects.

Faith, who we met earlier, reiterates this point:

> Do not dismiss the medical menopause ... I did, to my peril, which was understandable due to all the other operations/treatments etc. In fact, it was never even mentioned to me other than in a very quick conversation at the very beginning.
>
> I've struggled so much since treatment ended and I think a lot of this was actually menopausal. 100 per cent advocate for yourself to see a specialist regarding this when you are ready.

Go armed with information and fill out a symptom diary (such as the free Balance app), and explain the treatment you've had. It is so important to manage these symptoms for so many reasons, especially if you find yourself entering the perimenopausal or menopausal stage earlier than anticipated.

Menopause – what can I do to help myself?

Lifestyle advice is paramount for the management of menopause in addition to medication and other treatments. This includes:

- **General measures** (especially to help hot flushes and night sweats):
  - Avoid overdressing, wear light, cotton clothing and light colours.
  - Wash and clean skin regularly.
  - Use antiperspirants and use plain unscented face powder to absorb sweat.
  - Use a fan and avoid hot temperatures if possible. Leave windows open at night. Sleep with a thin sheet.
  - Use ice packs, eat cool foods, suck on ice chips or cold flannels.
  - Avoid triggers – keep a diary of what makes symptoms worse.
- **Dietary advice:**
  - Avoid spicy foods, caffeinated drinks and chocolate, which can increase hot flushes.
  - Stay hydrated.
  - Eat small regular meals.

- **Exercise:** this is a really important aspect when it comes to the treatment of menopause. We've already seen so many of the health benefits of exercise, but the benefits in relation to the menopause include a reduction in symptoms – especially of hot flushes, mood disturbance, brain fog, and insomnia. Exercise also offers a reduction in osteoporosis risk through weight-bearing exercises, as well as a reduction in cardiovascular risk. If you already exercise, it's important to change and 'shake up' your exercise routine. Studies have shown that a variety and combination of exercises is the most effective strategy to help manage a healthy weight during menopause, as well as managing the physical and psychological symptoms. The different exercise modalities include:
  - Aerobic exercise where the heart rate is raised – this includes activities such as swimming, brisk walking (so you're building up a sweat), cycling, rowing, running and high-intensity exercise classes.
  - Weight-bearing exercises reduce your risk of osteoporosis. These type of exercises encompass any 'exercise where you are on your feet and adding an additional force or jolt through your skeleton', according to the Royal Osteoporosis Society. This could include walking, dancing, gardening, tennis or other racquet sports, skipping, or climbing the stairs. Aim to do this two or three times a week.
  - Strength training to improve muscle mass which wanes as we age and go through menopause. Muscle strengthening exercises are movements where you move your muscles against resistance. This includes the use of resistance bands, weights or exercises such as press ups, where you lift your own body weight. Try to include two sessions of this a week.
  - Yoga or Pilates – helps with strength, balance, flexibility, relaxation, relieves aches and pains and can help with the pelvic floor.
  - Pelvic floor exercises – something that can be difficult to remember daily but they are vital for bladder, bowel and sexual function, as discussed in Chapter 12.
- **Sleep:** around 40 per cent of women complain of insomnia. Lack of sleep can negatively impact recovery from treatment, but also recovery from exercise. It also can make menopausal symptoms

worse. It is true that HRT can help with insomnia but is also worthwhile noting that practising good sleep hygiene will help manage the symptoms of menopause and recovery. Please see the Appendix for more on sleep hygiene.

- **Alcohol and smoking:** alcohol and smoking both increase the incidence of hot flushes. We also know that some may turn to drinking more alcohol as they feel so awful, despite the fact that alcohol is a depressant in itself, so can affect mood further.
- **CBT – Cognitive Behavioural Therapy:** a reduction in stress can reduce symptoms, especially hot flushes, sexual concerns, insomnia, aches and pains as well as helping with mood disorders.
- **Stress reduction:** this can reduce hot flushes through a combination of relaxation techniques which may include CBT, mindfulness, breathing exercises and yoga (see Useful Resources).
- **Acupuncture:** some individuals find acupuncture beneficial although there is no strong medical evidence as yet regarding its benefit.

Hormone Replacement Therapy or HRT

This medication offers a variety of benefits, including a reduction in symptoms and an increase in quality of life and well being, as well as a reduction in osteoporosis and cardiovascular risk.

HRT is made of oestrogen (which combats many of the symptoms experienced through the menopause), and progesterone (which protects the lining of the womb against the effects of oestrogen and keeps the lining thin).

There is a wide array of HRT available – patches, gels, sprays and tablets, as well as the Mirena coil, which can act as the progesterone component of HRT. There are also body-identical preparations out there which are better tolerated with fewer side effects and fewer risks. These preparations have a similar structure to naturally occurring hormones in the body.

Dr Stewart highlights that some women often question whether HRT is safe to take after CRC. Indeed, it is safe to take in those with colorectal cancer (as the cancer is not hormone sensitive unlike some breast cancers). It is best to talk to your family doctor or a doctor with a specialist interest in women's health to find the right initial preparation for you. Doses may need to be altered and the preparation or type of HRT changed till you find something that works for you. This is not unusual, so please don't give up if it doesn't work at first.

Management of specific symptoms

Genitourinary syndrome of menopause – 'My vagina and vulva feel like sandpaper: constantly itching, burning and dry'

(Also known as vulvovaginal atrophy or atrophic vaginitis.) This is where low oestrogen levels cause thinning, drying and inflammation of the vulva and vaginal walls. It can lead to an array of symptoms:

- Burning or itching in the vulva or vagina
- Vaginal discharge
- Urinary symptoms such as needing the toilet frequently, or urgently, burning when urinating, urine infections and incontinence, irritation in the vulval region and the vagina
- Pain during sexual intercourse
- Reduction in arousal or ability to orgasm
- Vaginal bleeding or bleeding after sex.

Treatment should include the following:

- Avoid douching and feminine products or soaps. Wash with plain water.
- Use vaginal moisturizers and water-based lubricants such as the Yes range or Replens. I often mention to women that just as one moisturizer might not suit your face and you try another, the same applies for vaginal moisturizers.
- Use a topical oestrogen as maintenance. Evidence shows the condition is progressive so the earlier you use topical oestrogen, the better the outcome and long-term management – so treat early!
- HRT – Ospemifene is new on the market, has an oestrogen-like effect on local tissues, and can be used in those with moderate to severe symptoms who are not candidates for oestrogen therapy.

Low libido – 'I just don't feel like having sex!'

Low libido can be due to a combination of psychological and physical issues. Hormonally, it is related to low oestrogen and testosterone. Once oestrogen has been replaced via HRT, if symptoms of low libido persist, a trial of testosterone gel can be used. Other symptoms of testosterone deficiency may include brain fog and poor concentration, tiredness and low energy, reduced bone density and low mood. Again, all should be treated with oestrogen first, before adding in testosterone (cream or gel) later on if symptoms persist. Sex therapy or psychosexual counselling is also an option to explore if symptoms have a psychological element as a result of trauma.

If you are unable to take HRT for any reason or it doesn't suit you, there are other medical options available on top of the lifestyle advice above. These include clonidine (for hot flushes), gabapentin or pregabalin (which can help with sleep and hot flushes), and antidepressants (which can help with mood disturbances and hot flushes).

The long and short of the menopause is that there is plenty that can be done so please don't hesitate to seek help (see Useful Resources).

Fertility

Having discussions regarding fertility should happen in a timely manner when it comes to your treatment, ideally with a fertility specialist. Potentially difficult decisions have to be made regardless of whether you are in a relationship or not as to whether you think you may wish to have children in the future. There is no shadow of a doubt that this is a double hit along with a cancer diagnosis and the pain that can tag along with it. But being informed about your options at the time and for the future can help some way in taking back control.

There are many aspects surrounding fertility preservation to consider: the stage at diagnosis, how much time there is before the initiation of cancer treatment, what treatments will be undertaken, medical history, and so on. Many treatments are available in the UK on the NHS if you have had cancer, but this again can depend on various factors such as your postcode, age and whether you have had children in the past.

How can treatment affect fertility in men?

Bowel cancer surgery can cause erection and ejaculation problems, but sperm counts remain unaffected.

Radiotherapy for rectal cancers can potentially cause infertility as treatment is given around the pelvis area, therefore affecting sperm quality and counts.

Chemotherapy can slow down or stop the production of sperm temporarily or permanently. This is dependent on the drugs and doses of drugs involved. The more drugs a patient is on, the higher the chance of a reduced sperm count or no sperm count at all. If there is a temporary reduction, it can take several years to recover.

Sperm storage should be offered prior to treatment and in the UK funding on the NHS exists for this but it is dependent on where you live. Sperm can be stored up to 10 years or longer. Fertility specialists can give more information regarding this.

How can treatment affect fertility in women?

Pelvic radiotherapy often causes infertility. Radiotherapy can affect the uterus and may affect your chances of having a successful pregnancy after fertility treatment. Your healthcare team will explain your options, which may include surrogacy.

Chemotherapy can cause temporary or permanent infertility, and this is dependent on the drugs and doses used. Menstrual periods may continue, become irregular or stop during treatment. However, if your periods continue, it doesn't guarantee that you could become pregnant. If periods stop, they may return up to a year later. If it is more than a year since your last period, it may be that you are going through the menopause.

We know the younger the individual, the more likely periods will return and the more likely fertility will be preserved.

If, however, you face the prospect of infertility as a result of treatment, there are options – but it is crucial to understand that all options have varying success rates and will depend on a whole host of factors including the individual, their treatment for their cancer and the fertility preservation method they use.

Options to have children include:

Fertility preservation

Freezing eggs – if you do not have a partner yet, or do not want to use your current partner's sperm, then there is an option to freeze your eggs, which will be harvested after your ovaries are stimulated. These can be used at a later date with sperm. Egg freezing has a less successful pregnancy rate than freezing embryos.

Freezing embryos – the partner's sperm or the donor sperm can be used in a laboratory setting to fertilize harvested eggs from the female. This process forms an embryo which can then be frozen for use at a later date. At this point, the embryo would be introduced into the womb. The embryos are the joint property of the couples, so permission is needed from both parties to use them in the future.

Freezing ovarian tissue – otherwise known as ovarian tissue cryopreservation. This is not widely available, so please check the situation locally. A small piece of ovarian tissue is removed pre-treatment and frozen. It is put back into the body after treatment finishes and, if it starts working again, eggs may be produced from the ovary.

Ovarian suppression

A GnRH analogue such as zoladex can be given to suppress the ovaries during treatment every 3–4 weeks. It shifts the female body essentially into a 'medical menopause' so the side effects are those of menopause. The hope is that, when treatment has finished and the GnRH analogue is stopped, the ovaries are no longer suppressed and ovulation and egg release may occur once more with preserved fertility. This is not suitable for all, nor does it work for everyone.

IVF

This is the process by which egg production is stimulated by daily injection of hormones. These are then harvested and collected as above and also as above can either be frozen as eggs or frozen as embryos.

Donor eggs or sperm

Sperm or eggs donated to a sperm bank or egg bank can be used for future embryo formation.

Surrogacy

This is where a person carries and gives birth to a baby for another person or couple. Full surrogacy is where the eggs of the intended mother or a donor are used and there is therefore no genetic connection between the baby and the surrogate. Partial surrogacy (also known as straight or traditional surrogacy) involves the surrogate's egg being fertilized with the sperm of the intended father. Ensure you register with licensed fertility clinics if going down this route. See the Surrogacy UK website, or your local organizations if you live outside the UK.

Adoption or fostering

For further information see the British Adoption and Fostering Academy website or a local site if you live outside the UK.

This is not an easy decision to make and options are best discussed with a fertility specialist, who can give you a clearer idea about what would be most suitable, what the chances of success are, and what route to pursue. There is also more information regarding fertility treatments on the Human Fertilisation and Embryology Authority (HFEA) website.

It is important to note that contraception should be used for both men and women during radiotherapy and chemotherapy and for about a year after treatment ends. These treatments can damage sperm and eggs or harm a developing baby.

When it comes to receiving a diagnosis of early menopause and infertility, it can be psychologically crushing and cruel, and an immense grief may come during this period. It is really important to seek psychological help or support if needed to help you through this difficult time. Talk to friends or family if you can, and explain how you are feeling. Ask your doctor or specialist nurse to refer you to a counsellor or support group. And most of all, please don't bear this weight alone or in silence.

14

Scanxiety and surveillance

Risk of recurrence (cancer returning) – the topic no one really wants to ever talk about

I'm not going to talk facts and figures when it comes to talking about the risk of cancer recurrence, because we are not a statistic. We are individuals of varying ages, sexes and ethnicities, with different circumstances and medical histories, and different cancers.

When I was diagnosed with stage 3B rectal cancer, my mind flitted back to my med school days when I was taught the chances of surviving this stage of cancer at five years post-diagnosis were 50:50. Thankfully, medicine and treatments have come a long way in the 23 years since I was being lectured by the professor of colorectal surgery. I had quite frank discussions with my oncologist about my personal risk of recurrence or progression to stage 4 cancer. This is not for everyone; however, as a medic, I felt it was important to know, especially with the historic knowledge that I held. She delivered the stats to me cautiously, with a caveat that to this day has stuck with me. The survival studies performed were in older, often male, Caucasian individuals and so this data may not translate to a young Asian female in her late thirties who is fit and healthy with no genetic cause identified. So yes, there is a theoretical risk, but no one can hand on their heart quantify this. So, I'll reiterate again, you are not a number.

Fear of recurrence or disease progression – 'I'm scared'

This doesn't mean you're not frightened of cancer recurrence. For a while, fleeting thoughts of recurrence would pass through my mind with every cough, every stomach ache and even when a strange skin rash developed. The whirlwind of emotions, soon escalating to a

191

tornado, but my medical brain kicking into action, saying 'let's wait and see, it's just a cold right now'.

The first year after a cancer diagnosis can bring intense and uncomfortable feelings where your mind is swept away into the 'what ifs?'. I found the more time that elapsed from diagnosis, the more the intensity of emotions dampened and the safer I felt, but let's be clear, I was still petrified during scan season. The more time that passes with clear scans, the better the chances of five-year survival. That is a medical fact. But I've learnt from my own diagnosis that anything can change at any given moment. So, I try to choose to live in the moment. The here and now.

How do you live with the fear of the cancer potentially returning?

It has been estimated that one- to two-thirds of cancer patients worry about the fear of recurrence, so you are not alone. This loss of control can also make you feel vulnerable and see your emotions spiralling.

Tips: Managing the fear of recurrence

- Acceptance – it is a normal reaction to worry, and it is so important to acknowledge that worry as well. It is ok to feel scared, and this may lessen over time.
- Know your surveillance schedule (see below) – knowing you are under surveillance and having a robust and thorough follow-up plan can help reduce the fear of recurrence by giving you back some control.
- Know the symptoms of cancer recurrence to help you feel more in control (see below) – although recurrence of cancer can present just on routine surveillance scans, it is also important to know the signs or symptoms of recurrence and, if concerned, discuss this with a doctor or your cancer nurse specialist.
- What triggers you? Cancerversaries, anniversaries, scan times, appointments, new symptoms? Know your triggers so you can best anticipate and prepare for the surge in emotions.
- Take control where you can – no one wants to be in this position, but take back the reins by ensuring you look after your health, attend appointments, and be body aware, letting a doctor know of any concerns.

Many of the tips I share in the 'scanxiety' section below will also help you manage the uncertainty too. If the fear is persistently affecting you or affecting your quality of life and mood, please do contact your doctor.

Potential symptoms of recurrence – 'What do I need to look for?'

In my opinion, it is imperative to know what signs and symptoms patients with cancer should be looking out for. This is something that has been voiced to me out of concern by bowel cancer patients. They felt this wasn't often discussed after treatment so they weren't fully informed or equipped to know when to seek help.

What you should know is that if a symptom is persistent, it is worth mentioning to your doctor or CNS. The most common site of recurrence is in the liver or lung. Recurrence in the bowel is less common if surgery was deemed successful, unless you have certain genetic conditions.

If you have had bowel surgery, there is a chance you will have a 'new normal' bowel habit, and ironically many of the symptoms can mimic those of bowel cancer. However, if there is a change away from this new bowel habit that is ongoing, persistent, or if you are worried, it is worth checking.

Potential symptoms of cancer recurrence in your bowel include:

- Any bleeding from your bottom or stoma that does not go away and persists for more than two weeks
- A change in your bowel habit that persists for more than three weeks
- Any unexplained loss of weight, lack of appetite and/or a constant feeling of nausea
- Extreme and increasing fatigue or lethargy
- Pain in your tummy which is severe, or lasts more than two weeks or is associated with abdominal swelling/vomiting/not passing stool or wind.

Potential symptoms to be aware of if cancer has spread to the liver:

- Discomfort or pain on the right side of your abdomen.
- Itchy skin

- Nausea
- Unexplained weight loss and poor appetite
- Swelling of the abdomen (called ascites)
- Yellowing of the skin and eyes (jaundice).

Potential symptoms if cancer has spread to your lungs:

- Persistent cough
- Feeling breathless
- Recurrent chest infections
- Coughing up blood
- Chest pain.

Remember there are many other medical conditions that can cause these symptoms. Either way, they should be discussed with your doctor so they can decide what investigations may be needed.

Surveillance

Surveillance is a term used for following up with colorectal cancer patients, to allow early detection of local recurrence or metastases (spread of the cancer to other places in the body away from the bowel), without any symptoms.

Bowel cancer surveillance schedules vary from country to country and slightly between hospitals. It will also depend on the stage at which your cancer was diagnosed. It is important to check with your cancer specialist nurse or your medical team what surveillance programme you will be offered so you are in the know and have a plan for follow up to ensure you're being checked at regular intervals, to hopefully give you some peace of mind, control and space to breathe.

What does surveillance potentially involve?

For those that have had curative treatment, surveillance may include the following investigations at varying intervals deemed appropriate by your hospital and following NICE guidance.

This may include:

- **CEA (carcinoembryonic antigen):** this is a blood test for a tumour marker called CEA. This seems to be more helpful in surveillance if it was elevated at diagnosis. Necessity and frequency of tests will be determined by your hospital.
- **CT scan of the chest, abdomen (tummy area) and pelvis:** this is looking for any spread of disease which, as we discussed earlier, may occur in the liver and lungs, as well as in the lining of the abdomen (peritoneum).
- **Colonoscopy at varying intervals:** usually at one year post diagnosis and then another three years after the last colonoscopy, in the UK.

Follow-up appointments also involve consultations with your surgical or oncological team, via your cancer specialist colorectal nurse. They will ask about how you're managing with side effects and in the longer term post treatment and surgery, with bowel dysfunction, and then of course asking if you have any worrying symptoms, and arranging any necessary tests if they are concerned, even if that falls outside your surveillance schedule.

With four-monthly CEA blood checks and six-monthly CT scans for the first two years, I felt that I lived life between scans. Never wanting to plan much till the next scan was done. An 'NED' (no evidence of disease, or a clear scan with no evidence of recurrence or spread to liver and lungs) gave you a green light to start living and breathing again – until the next time. I found this way of living exhausting in the early days, so I found a toolkit to help manage the scanxiety, which I'll talk about below. The build-up, the worrying, the angst, the anxiety and then the crescendo – the result. The permission to process another milestone. You've survived, you've made it!

Since going on to yearly follow-up, I'm definitely more at peace. I know that might not feel comfortable for a lot of people but for me, it gives me a longer time to breathe and to live, rather than waiting in fear, worrying that the next scan is coming up. In my case, the team have made a decision to continue surveillance (in view of my young age at diagnosis and the nature of the disease at diagnosis).

I live by the mantra that no news is good news; foolhardy for some, I'm sure, but a protective mechanism that allows me to live and actually get in some living, despite all that has happened. Of course, when I have run into any difficulty relating to my health, I feel empowered and know exactly where to go to seek help, to hopefully alleviate any concerns early on, and I too have had scares.

If you are on life long treatment, the frequency and type of investigations will be governed by your oncologist. and the treatment schedules in place to establish whether there is any disease regression, stability or progression, which will can help determine the next plan of action.

Scanxiety

Scanxiety is the apprehension and worry experienced by a patient who has or has had cancer, whilst waiting for a scan to take place or for a scan result.

The letter lands on your doormat; the hospital stamp is instantly recognizable. The envelope. The writing. It starts. Adrenaline pumps furiously. It's time. That dreaded scan time. The box of uncertainty flies open. The scan you so want to tell you that you're ok. The scan you also don't want to have knowing it may bring absolute chaos and heartache once more.

As someone who never wishes time away, I would give anything for time to pass during and around scan time, to know that I'm still free of cancer or with no disease progression.

So here, described below, is my first experience of scanxiety. At the time of my diagnosis, there was no time to process or even realize what was truly going on as I was whisked from one scan to the next. Up until this point, I had never experienced this phenomenon.

It was my first scan since diagnosis. And I'd kept this one under my hat. That fear. Again, of the unknown.

I was told after diagnosis that at some point, I would be required to have a scan of my liver. On my original CT back in September, the day they found my cancer, they found a couple of 'spots on my liver'. At the time three different radiologists had looked at my scan and felt, on balance, that these were not deposits of cancer, thankfully. However, later down the line, there was a U turn. One that left us shaken. They felt I would need another MRI to characterize the 'spots' in further detail, just to double check they were non-cancerous.

When they told me, I ran out of the room. After my last two MRIs, the claustrophobia I had already mildly suffered with prior to diagnosis was somewhat magnified and even more traumatic. The irrational side of my brain took over and I knew there was no way they would chivvy me into the MRI scanner again – unless I was heavily sedated or, in fact, they could arrange for it to be carried out in an open air scanner. I remembered that at the initial diagnosis, my husband practically had his head in the scanner with me. To the point where I'm surprised the top of his brain didn't show up on my scans!

After further discussions, it was agreed an ultrasound might suffice on this occasion, so I attended hospital again for the necessary examination.

I had swept the fact that I needed one under the carpet.

But in the week running up to the scan, the anxiety crept back in, precious sleep became scant and I withdrew, feeling overwhelmed, facing the reality of my 'new normal' of scans and scanxiety. Of this life between scans. Of waiting. Of worrying about recurrence or disease progression. Of catastrophizing. Of the reality of the potential for cancer to rear its ugly head once again.

On scan day, my husband was thankfully allowed in the room with me as the consultant radiologist skilfully manoeuvred her probe around my liver. As we all held our breath, and through mindless banter, she finally divulged what I so needed to hear. 'It's not cancer.' Thankfully the 'liver lesions' were just liver cysts, non-cancerous fluid-filled sacs on the liver that are common and will cause no harm.

As CT scans are part of bowel cancer surveillance – usually CT scans of the chest, abdomen and pelvis – the scanxiety that reigns can become intrusive for many, impacting day-to-day life. Impacting work, family life, and relationships as irrational thoughts kick in. Everyone else's worries seem trivial whilst you feel consumed by the worry of your fate.

What I will say from experience is this. Everyone differs in how they react around scan time, how they deal with the stress it causes and the wait for the results. They also tend to develop their own coping mechanisms, which is really important and very individual.

I found six-monthly CT scans hard going from the moment the letter arrived on my doorstep with a time and date to the time I was told I had a clear scan. One would think you would be overjoyed with an NED result (No Evidence of Disease) but there were times it felt like an anticlimax. I don't want to sound ungrateful, but at times I felt void of any further emotion, having been through the mill in the weeks preceding the scan, and waiting for results, and I was, quite frankly, frazzled. What it did give me, however, was permission to breathe again and, after a couple of scans, I did decide to mark the occasion by doing something special, celebrating or treating myself! Of course, this is not for everyone, but it did become more and more important as the children grew older and started understanding the implications of scans. We would always say it was for a check-up but as they grew older and developed more understanding, further questions would arise. 'Is it checking for the cancer coming back, Mummy?' We've always believed in protecting the children but also in being honest with them. So, they also now get involved with these milestones, including clear scans and celebrations to mark these moments, allowing us to continue moving forwards as a family. Once, my son insisted with celebrating with doughnuts... I was thinking more of champagne!

Continuing from this, it is important to recognize that scanxiety can also infiltrate those around you, and loved ones, who may feel the palpable angst too. Although you may not feel in the best position to support them yourself, with your own burdensome worry, it is worth making sure they are looking after themselves and have others to talk to during this time. So, what can we do to manage the uncertainty that goes hand in hand with scanxiety? These tips may not apply to everyone and don't necessarily dissipate all the fear, but maybe can help make it more manageable. So here we go:

Tips: Dealing with scanxiety

- Know yourself around scan time – know how you react to stress/anxiety and what helps you. For example, I now see a pattern of behaviour changes. I find my job more difficult, I'm more irritable, less tolerant and suffer insomnia and panic at night while going into overdrive and over distracting in the day. I have little headspace. Fun mum gets a little lost. I have been told I have more of a 'cement face' as a friend put it, and I feel utterly exhausted and consumed.
- Distraction – is key. I tend to work more: more awareness work, throwing myself into the positives cancer gave me, exercising more, and keeping time filled up. I make dates with friends and family and often book spontaneous memory-making events in a bid to remind myself I'm still here and living. My family and friends have had some fabulous trips out fuelled by my scanxiety, and my wardrobe has gained some choice items!
- Share your feelings with loved ones, someone you trust, or a counsellor. Share with work colleagues when the time comes if it helps. I'm lucky to work with colleagues who are sympathetic, although

I'm sure they won't always fully comprehend. What I do feel by communicating this is that it helps me 'just be' during a time where my behaviour may change. I may be quieter, less animated and more withdrawn. Explain what those around you might do to help (because remember they can't feel everything you are feeling). And be honest.

- Consult your team – let the radiology team or your cancer team know if you are prone to claustrophobia so they can take extra measures and give extra time to talk you through the process. Take someone with you to the scan (although during CT scans, no one can come into the actual room due to the radiation risks). You could also ask for a small dose of sedative beforehand if you are really struggling – discuss this further with your doctor.
- Talk to others who have trodden a similar path – whether that be online, face to face or through a support group, it can make you feel less alone and even less scared. I know as the years go by, I draw much of my strength during scan time from the online community, and I'm so grateful for this.
- Try to live for the moment – easier said than done. Try to immerse yourself in mindful activities/mindfulness, even if they are active in nature. I know for me, personally, sitting and listening to apps did not help me relax. I choose to take nature walks and to cook, for example. Anything that helps you focus on the here and now.
- Know it's ok to not be ok – it's ok to be scared. Try to set limits to the time you think and worry, maybe write down these thoughts. Journal.
- Plan something to look forward to after the scan, or treat yourself. That new perfume, that new golf club, a new haircut, dinner with friends. Whatever works for you.
- Have a mantra – for me this was, 'Look how far you have come.'
- Practise breathing exercises/meditation. There are some examples of this in Chapter 16.
- Look after your mental health – see Chapter 16.
- And of course, as always, look after yourself, by exercising, eating well and trying to maintain a good sleep routine.

You will find your own pattern. And although scans never get easier, as time goes by, I am able to now put my lifejacket on quietly, and put strategies into place to help me stay afloat and manage the best I can.

And remember with each scan that passes, just look how far you've come.

15

The emotional burden of cancer

'Everything is hard, before it is easy.'

Goethe

The emotional burden of cancer really is a minefield. I never knew you could experience so many different emotions within a 24-hour period. Tears one minute, laughter the next. It was, and still is at times, all-consuming.

How the burden is carried indeed varies between individuals and is dependent on so many factors: personality type, coping strategies, the cancer, stage and treatment proposed, social set-up, family and friends' support, outlook on life, whether there are pre-existing physical or mental health problems, and so forth.

This chapter looks at some of the emotions experienced after a diagnosis of cancer. Not everyone experiences all of them and they may differ in intensity depending on where you are within your treatment or your surveillance pathway.

Firstly, let's look at grief and the grief cycle. Why? Because looking back, these are some of the very first emotions I experienced when the words 'you've got cancer' were spoken.

Grief

From the time of diagnosis, I would flit from a state of shock and denial to utter sadness, oblivious to the fact that I would also be grieving for the life I knew before cancer (BC) too. Grief can occur for the loss of body parts, a limb, a breast, and I certainly do miss my previous bowel function, so on that level, I do miss half my rectum and part of my colon too. Giving yourself time and permission to grieve is an essential part of the healing process, as is recognizing that a grief reaction is a normal reaction to a cancer diagnosis.

Stages of grief were identified by psychiatrist Elisabeth Kübler-Ross back in 1969. These may be familiar to you: denial, anger, bargaining, sadness and depression, and acceptance.

Learning about these stages can help you try to make sense of these emotions that may come with this diagnosis (often in any order). Remembering that grief does not have a timeline can help us understand why, sometimes, feelings of grief can wax and wane when we least expect them.

Denial

Denial helps us switch into survival mode. The feeling of numbness and shock almost helps one cope with the initial stage after you find out you have cancer. I fear I initially spent most of my time after diagnosis in the denial phase, so the stages such as anger and bargaining were less of a feature of my grief till later on. Probably even before diagnosis, in my mind, I wouldn't even entertain thoughts of being sick, let alone having cancer. I became very detached and depersonalized from my diagnosis and saw myself as an outsider going through all the necessary motions, investigations and treatment as part of the course. I spent a long time disbelieving this was actually happening to me, to the point I didn't ever read one of the letters from my specialists. Eighteen months on from diagnosis, I was asked during trauma-based cognitive behavioural therapy to read each and every single letter and go through details with a fine toothcomb, as a way of processing the traumatic event, in a bid to search for acceptance that, indeed, I had had cancer.

Anger

Anger is a normal emotion and part of your fight or flight instinct. Some people may manifest this in the usual shouting and ranting, but I found mine would manifest in low tolerance levels and irritability.

I found I rarely felt angry on receipt of my cancer diagnosis. Rarely did I think 'Why me?', but when I did, it was vented as more of a frustration – 'Why do my family and I have to go through this?' 'Why are my family affected?' 'Why does everyone else get to carry on with their lives?', rather than pity for myself. It felt so unfair and unjust – as a younger person, I didn't fit the bill for a cancer diagnosis. When I finished treatment, comments like 'at least you're done now, just forget about it' would also ignite anger.

I found that anger manifested usually on the dark days, around scan time, during difficulties in treatment when I felt the world carrying on without me. Interestingly, the anger was actually worse after I finished treatment, when all I wanted to do was to go back to a normal which was no more.

I was angry that my body had been floored, and there was a long road ahead, my destination unclear.

I was angry that I was a mess and felt ineffectual – I just couldn't do anything well – be it parenting, being a wife, or working, to the ability I could pre-cancer.

I felt that cancer still had me in a vice, and I was angry that I no longer had a life I recognized. My life before cancer. That carefree, cancer-free life, where I needn't live in fear. Even my old bowel function, I missed it, and felt angry that I missed out on meals, events or time with my loved ones as, in the early days, I would spend most of the time in the toilet or traipsing back and forth from the toilet.

I was furious some days with those around me who seemed inherently ungrateful for their first world problems; they hadn't changed, but I had. And so friendships inadvertently changed because of my new perspective, until I was able to adjust to my 'new normal'. I felt anger when people moaned about getting older – in my head ageing is a privilege, and if I was lucky enough to see my next birthday cancer-free – well, happy days.

On reflection, I was in a sorry state mentally.

It is worthwhile mentioning that often, lurking behind the anger, are a hundred different emotions (frustration, disappointment, anxiety, embarrassment, shame, low self-confidence and esteem) longing to be unpicked, and if they are not, an explosion may ensue, where a trivial matter causes an outburst from nowhere.

Anger is only problematic if you find it is affecting your mood, is persistent, is disproportionate to the situation, if you become aggressive and threatening towards others, or if it is directed at the wrong people. If this is the case, please see a doctor to get help.

Bargaining

When we are in pain, it is difficult to accept that we cannot change things. Guilt often accompanies this emotion, which we'll look at shortly.

If only I had gone to the doctor earlier. If only I had been referred earlier. If only I hadn't smoked, had drunk less alcohol, exercised more. If only my mother didn't have a genetic form of cancer. If only I hadn't eaten all that charred red meat.

Of course, it is natural to think 'if only'. The reality is we can't change the past, and we need to conserve our energy for the here and now and moving forwards. These questions are often unanswerable and so best left alone.

It can be a struggle to find the meaning behind why cancer happened but often reaching out, talking, and sharing one's story with open dialogues may be helpful.

Sadness and depression

It is really important to distinguish between sadness and depression. Sadness may be a normal response to a cancer diagnosis. I found this often ebbed and flowed, related to how tired or ill I felt. On the other hand, depression is pervasive and interferes with everyday activities, quality of life and recovery. It can require professional help.

This phase can witness feelings of overwhelm, low energy levels and helplessness.

Was I ever depressed? Actually, what I did feel at times was a deep sadness – but only momentarily crossing the threshold into depression, for a few weeks. I'll talk more about this when we discuss mental health further.

Acceptance

This doesn't necessarily mean you're absolutely fine and have 'let go' of what has happened. For me, it means I can sit comfortably, most of the time, with cancer and the aftermath; the pain mentally has lessened with time, and I have come to peace with it. It also meant that I could go on to make a new plan for life, exploring options and avenues that I might not have entertained previously.

With cancer, eventually there has to be a level of acceptance as Danni, our psychotherapist, tells me, and it's important for individuals to be able to 'accept the circumstance in that moment. Accept where you are. Don't fight it or resist. It doesn't mean you are submissive towards your cancer and often those that manage to accept that cancer came to make its mark, are more likely to positively be able to move forward, further on down the line.'

Grief can manifest at any time, much like one may feel waves of grief on the birthday of a loved one who has died, and feelings may be evoked once more during cancer milestones such as cancerversaries or scan times. These feelings can temporarily come flooding back in no particular order once more.

Guilt

Guilt forms part of the rainbow of emotions that follows a cancer diagnosis, treatment, and life after cancer. It doesn't manifest every day and tends to come and go as it pleases, but when it does, it can become quite intrusive.

> **7 December 2018, night before cycle 2 of chemo**
> ROUND 2: DING DING!
> 4 a.m.
> Here we are.
> Can't sleep.
> Now I know what's coming, I think it's harder than the unknown last cycle? I'm not sure. Either way, it's happening. And I'm scared.
> As are my family. My six-year-old daughter asked me two days ago, 'When does chemo start?' And she burst out crying when I told her. 'Mummy, I don't want you to have it, I don't want you to be ill again.' Because they lose their mother, albeit temporarily. It's so confusing for them, as I partially recover from each hurdle, to then become pretty much bed bound for a period of time after the next treatment/procedure.
> And my mother. I can hear the panic and worry in her voice as she desperately tries to keep it together, offering me anything and everything to try to make me feel better.
> Then there is my rock, my husband, who loses his wife to a bubble of fatigue and fragility. But he continues to lovingly mop up my tears, attends to every random food craving I have, and sits quietly with me, just 'being there', as I exist. Cancer comes loaded with guilt at times, especially for my loved ones, having to go through all this. Having to watch me in disarray, a total mess. It's not fair. There I said it. I sound like a toddler not getting their own way, but it's just not. Hopefully this time will be different, with the dose reduction of drugs. But for now, we need to damage control as best we can.

During counselling, I talked about guilt A LOT. Below is a list I wrote of all of the things I felt guilty about, which I then read out to Danni, my therapist:

- Guilt that my children and husband missed out on time as a family or with me, and still sometimes do (usually around scan times where I become preoccupied mentally)
- Guilt that the children still sometimes had to 'just get on with it' as I was beyond exhausted some days
- Guilt that my parents had to witness their daughter see such suffering
- Guilt that I became a burden
- Guilt that I have myriad post-treatment side effects which only occasionally irritate me but actually I should be just grateful that treatment has worked for now
- Guilt that I developed sciatica which stopped me doing some activities with the children and they still had to help me
- Guilt that everyone has been so wonderful to my family, given us so much time, care and attention and I will never be able to pay them back
- Guilt that I feel unable to pull my weight at home some days
- Guilt that I'm struggling to return to work in a linear manner
- Guilt that I look fine
- Guilt that I'm not always fine
- Guilt that the school teacher told me my son's performance did drop a little while I was in treatment, but picked up in subsequent weeks
- Guilt that now my family has a 'family history' possibly increasing their lifetime risk of colorectal cancer
- Guilt that I should be eating a super-healthy fibre-rich diet to reduce my risk of cancer recurrence, but all I can face eating during chemotherapy is a Rich Tea biscuit
- And finally an irrational guilt that cancer came knocking at our door and it turned our life upside down.

So, what did we do, and what can you do?

Guilt usually occurs when there has been harm caused (intentionally or unintentionally), and encourages humans to 'do the right thing'. People have different thresholds for experiencing guilt depending on their moral compass and the situation at hand. Let's be clear – cancer was not caused by anyone, and is certainly not anyone's fault. What we need to remember is that the past cannot be changed and what happens at a cellular level cannot be controlled ... Dwelling on the past continues to reinforce the negative and heighten the feelings of self-blame.

Yet as someone who has had cancer, we can use this emotion to punish ourselves for the impact that our diagnosis has had on others. And the sadness and remorse we may feel towards the 'wrongdoing' can preoccupy the mind. I was reminded by Danni that guilt in this situation is a wasted emotion. And I'm here reminding you to be kind and compassionate to yourself, as what you are experiencing is emotionally depleting as it is.

As best as I could, I tried to stay positive, thankful, and rationalize these emotions, sometimes looking back at just how far all of us had come and the positives that cancer in some way gave us. I'll talk more of this gratitude later on. And I tried to identify the emotions behind the guilt, such as anger, sadness and vulnerability. For example, I'm usually the main carer to my children and I felt great sadness and frustration that I just couldn't do it, and in fact not only did I feel guilt, I felt envious of others taking them out, spending time that I couldn't offer. I felt angry they lost their mother figure, and I was constantly worried how they were coping, yet I knew they were being lovingly and well looked after by those around me. Recognizing these emotions helps process the guilt and nudge it to the side, saving energy for where it is needed.

If you find yourself feeling this way, in any situation, writing down your feelings and challenging them, and exploring the reasons behind them can be helpful.

Finally, ask yourself, if your loved one during cancer treatment and beyond told you all the reasons they were feeling guilty, what would you say to them?

'Talk to yourself as you would someone you love.'

Survivor's guilt

Survivor's guilt is a particular type of guilt that develops in those that have survived a life-threatening event. Some feel guilty they survived while others died. I felt this when those people I had bonded with through cancer later had disease progression or in fact died. Why did I survive?

Survivor's guilt is a well-recognized response to trauma, even if it can feel irrational, and it may be a symptom of PTSD. People with survivor's guilt should try to acknowledge these feelings and allow time to process the grief and trauma. This may include therapy. They also might find it beneficial to help others in some way to help alleviate their feelings. This may be through raising awareness, making a charitable donation, working with a charity donating blood or lending support to others.

Self-esteem/self-confidence/self-image

'Look at what your body and mind got you through.'

I really hadn't appreciated how much a cancer diagnosis and its treatment could impact one's self-worth, self-esteem, self-confidence and self-image. Although an extrovert I, too, like many, have my insecurities. These seemed to be magnified and I felt like a shell of the person I was before cancer, coming out of treatment. Your self-image may change due to the physical and emotional changes that cancer brings, and this in turn can affect your confidence.

Somewhere along the line, I also lost confidence in my body's ability to stay cancer free, be pain free, to have controlled bowel function, and to emotionally be in a stable and rational place.

I found it perturbing and unsettling not being able to do much to the best of my ability.

I would worry about my ability to exercise, to go out, to even go away for the weekend due to the fear something would go wrong and my body wouldn't cope, and I struggled with 'firsts' – first long hike, first weekend away with friends, first holiday – because I no longer trusted my body. Yet what a powerhouse it was, to have got me through the previous taxing months.

Body image

Physical changes to the body affect body image (thoughts about how we feel and think about how our body looks and what we think others see), which in turn can impact self-image (your thoughts about yourself). Alongside self-image, body image can be affected. I eventually put on weight with the steroids and inactivity during chemo and my hair thinned, and my face looked tired, but others never let on if they noticed, and often I was told I looked 'normal'. In fact, I fretted that I looked reasonably 'normal' on the outside, but everything on the inside had changed and felt far from comfortable, and actually that people just wouldn't understand as a result how I was feeling. I also struggled to look at my scars, let alone touch them. Not so much because I was embarrassed but more that it was a reminder of what had indeed happened.

Your body image can take a hit through treatment as your body changes due to the effects of treatment or cancer. Weight changes, hair loss, stomas, surgery scars, loss of a limb or organ, rashes from treatment, fatigue, loss of energy and sexual health problems. Some of these physical changes may improve as time passes; some will be permanent.

Tips: Body image

- Let your specialist team know that you are struggling, there may be suggestions of places for support or resources to help manage the changes.
- Let people support you.
- Give yourself time for a period of adjustment.
- Remind yourself daily what your body got you through and how far you've come. Sometimes, I felt like shutting myself away from the world, climbing under the covers and pretending I wasn't there, but every so often, I needed to remind myself of these things.
- Try therapy/counselling.
- Stay physically active, this will help you feel better about yourself and your body.

'I'm FINE'

'My mouth says I'm ok. My fingers say I'm fine. My heart says I'm broken.'

Unknown

I could probably leave this quote right there and I think it summarizes how we can so often portray ourselves – this need to give off the persona, that we've got this, we are coping and we have all our shit together. Why do we do this?

How many times a day or a week do you reply 'I'm fine' when someone enquires about your wellbeing?

Here's the real acronym for FINE:

F***ed up/freaked out
Insecure
Neurotic
Emotional

Danni suggested I stopped saying 'I'm fine' when I just wasn't. And persuaded me to stop saying 'I should be fine' when I clearly shouldn't. Why did I see not being ok as a weakness? To be vulnerable and feel fragile. People only had to look at me and I would feel myself crack.

What I did find, though, was that counselling became my safe place where I could truly be myself, and not be 'fine', let all my emotions go and get my emotional fix each week. I found this to be a crutch to see me through the week ahead.

Research from the Mental Health Foundation shows that only 19 per cent of people who say they are fine are in fact fine, leaving 81 per cent that aren't. And on average an adult will say 'I'm fine' 14 times a week. That was more like 14 times a day for me some days, because if I said it enough, I believed that I was.

So why did I say it?

- Because it made me feel that I had everything under control (when I actually hadn't always)
- Because I didn't want to burden others
- It's not always the right time to blurt out that actually you have 583 problems (for example on a school run). Who has the time?
- Because I was tired and fed up of feeling this way
- Because it can be ritualistic and polite
- Because people sometimes don't want to talk or open up
- Because it seems trivial (although you have feelings over it) or you think it will blow over.

What I learnt to do was show my vulnerability, rather than carry around a front that I felt people needed to see. So although I still may choose not to divulge my 583 problems on the school run, I am able to choose when and where to show my vulnerability, express that I may be struggling and ask for support.

Loneliness

I mentioned at the beginning that I really hoped this book would be a companion to you, a loved one, or carer, or just informative, giving an insight into cancer and the effects that ripple through an individual's life and their wider circle. The elephant in the room is this: I have never felt so alone in my entire life, yet I was blessed with the biggest army, best dream team and most loving family that I could ever ask for (who, let's be clear, are still the people who stand by my side day after day). However, it is tremendously difficult for people to understand the emotions one lives through each day. I also spent A LOT of time on my own, when feeling unwell or recovering, and although this is an essential part of treatment and recovery, I found my own thoughts to be toxic at times (fuelled by a cocktail of sleep deprivation, drugs, pain, frustration and loneliness and a lack of endorphins!).

May 2019

I've also struggled with loneliness and the sense of not wanting to burden my friends as time elapsed since my diagnosis and treatment. I've already had so much unconditional support, love, walks, lunches, therapy and treats. But it's amazing how an illness one has suffered can make you feel so alien to the out-side world. And the upset seeing the world carry on and your perception that everyone is busily being productive around you achieving so much as you strug-gle to even get through a day some days and wash your hair, and maybe even venture downstairs, can really mess with your head. Don't get me wrong, I'm utterly aware what I have achieved by getting through treatment. And making it through a day intact is an achievement in itself. It is important to acknowledge there are some VERY HARD days too. And I wish I didn't have to invest so much time into all the extra appointments and things I have to do to keep myself in check and on the straight and narrow through recovery.

Thankfully, these days are becoming less common and usually in isolation and I'm pretty sure sheer exhaustion has a part to play. Communication with friends and family is key, because if they don't know, how can they help or even just know to listen or be there? However, I do think it's natural to think your friends might tire of your personal rollercoaster. I'm like a box of chocolates … You never know what you're going to get!

And unless they have stood in my shoes, no one can quite comprehend the annihilation my body and mind have been through, and actually I don't think even I appreciated the turmoil treatment and cancer had on myself. This can further alienate you from those around you. I also have a different perspective from others after cancer, and I feel some days that no one would understand.

So what can help?

- **Family and friends.** Sometimes people don't realize you are feeling alone, they think everyone is rallying around and assume someone else may be popping in and the cancer patient doesn't want to burden anyone any further. So ask for help, let them know how you are feeling, and explain what you think you need – whether that is a walk, a cup of tea, a daily text to check in. Whatever you think can make you feel held.
- **Social media.** For all its faults, the power of using this as catharsis, and then connecting with others of all different ages and backgrounds, some with a drive to share their story, raise awareness and support each other, was incredibly powerful. I joined the cancer community on Instagram and found the world's biggest virtual hug. Using your own story is incredibly healing for many people. On the converse, if you don't want to share your story but find comfort by reading or supporting others, that can be equally powerful. Some, on the other hand, do not feel this is for them, they do not want to be associated with cancer, or be associated with anyone else with cancer, and feel no need to talk about it any more than they have to – that's ok, too.
- **Support groups.** Joining support groups or forums can help you feel that you belong somewhere, and becoming part of the Bowel Cancer UK family really did this for me. Support groups exist on social media – Facebook has groups for stage 4 colorectal cancer and LARS as well as charities that have forums and groups to join (see Useful Resources).
- **Faith.** Some people turn to their faith to talk about their feelings of isolation, and can feel more at peace.
- **Counsellor.** I talk about counselling frequently and I can't tell you how important this was for me. It allowed me to feel heard and seen when it came to walking a path that no one else around me was experiencing, with no filter and completely uncensored.

Anticipatory anxiety – 'What if?'

Speaking to my therapist Danni, she speaks openly about individuals' experiences with anticipatory anxiety. The constant 'What ifs?'.

What is important to remember is that the 'What if?' is a thought, not a reality. And dwelling on such thoughts can generate anxiety as we try to anticipate unknowns and uncertainties.

What can be more constructive is changing the narrative from 'What If?' to 'Even if'. For example, 'What if I develop complications from surgery?' can be changed to 'Even if I have surgery, I may not have complications, and if I do, I trust the surgical team to rectify these'.

It is also useful to learn to bring yourself back into the here and now, rather than the 'What if?'. A useful mantra to bring yourself back is 'All is good in this moment', and hopefully you will be able to appreciate where you are in that moment in time. For example, 'I am here at home with my husband, and my children are in bed and we are safe. All is good in this moment.' Another example Danni gives is when patients say, 'What if I die or the cancer comes back?' Danni would counteract this by saying, 'But at this moment, you are alive', bringing them back to the here and now.

Living on the edge

Whether you have just been diagnosed, are in treatment or out of treatment, you may be feeling despair and that you are, indeed, living on a cliff edge. From this vantage point, things can sometimes look bleak, and one can feel desperate. In fact, there were days where I was, frankly, broken.

The tension and strain when awaiting a diagnosis and then a plan of treatment are immense. Off the scale. So much so that time actually moves backwards. Every time someone approaches me telling me about their new diagnosis of cancer, I always try to explain, and reassure them that this in fact is the most difficult part in many ways, as you're held in limbo. The uncertainty, together with having to go through multiple tests in the hope of reaching an answer, which may include biopsies, scans, appointments, and then the multidisciplinary meeting. All this hopefully will offer information regarding the stage of the cancer and then a treatment plan going forward.

Once they have that under their belt, many people find themselves, in a state of preparation for military action, where the patient and those around them rally round in preparation for treatment to commence.

After treatment, these feelings subside a little, but every now and then, they can surface once more. This was an extract from my journal around six months post treatment ending.

It's not been an easy week. First time working three days back to back. Difficult, complex patients. Multiple lists of complaints. (Tricky when I only have 10 minutes and my brain feels on the go-slow.) Heavy load of cancer patients or relatives with problems due to their loved ones with cancer or cancer-related death. It's intense. Emotionally exhausted. Spent, and not much left to give. Running late constantly which I seldom do. Tears between patients. Tears with a patient. Lots going on at home. Stressful. Children repeatedly asking why God gave me cancer this week. Heart wrenching (we keep trying to tell them … he didn't!).

Fatigue which is plague-like. Truth.

Anxiety. Rocketing.

Feel like I keep falling off a horse. And desperately trying to climb back on.

Not seen counsellor in eight weeks. This was a mistake.

Feel like I'm constantly 'failing' at things. Feel like no one understands. And to be honest nor do I. Was grand a few days ago.

Situation currently: crash and burn. Overwhelmed.

School asked for cakes for a cake sale, I feel like they have asked me to sort out Brexit.

I'm meant to be walking the Seven Sisters and part of the South Downs Way together with friends tomorrow and maybe plan our next adventure. I'm not going to write how far we intend to walk to take the pressure off me trying to complete it. But worried I'll have to bail due to fatigue. Not feeling physically or mentally that grand right now. But I'm sure the fresh air and girlie therapy will do me the world of good! There is part of me, though, that is so anxious about going. I just want to feel like 'me' again.

I've added this here as a reminder that recovery is a long and ongoing process and that indeed things do take time, we can have blips and it's important to reach out. I did complete the 20-mile walk but I also had a chat with some of the girls with me, letting them know how I felt. Before that, they were oblivious to how I was feeling because I looked fine, but actually letting people know did alleviate some of my angst, something my therapist often signposted me to do.

With time, that incessant feeling of living on the edge does recede as you find your own way to take a step back from the edge, breathe, get busy living, and take in all the views.

16

Mental health – seeking help and self-care

'Breathe, darling, this is just a chapter. It's not your whole story.'

S.C. Lourie

You don't have to be at your lowest to seek help. Period.

And this is my biggest take home message. When I look back, for me, mental health issues started seeping out of the woodwork from day one. How can something so life changing not affect your mental health in some shape or form? Not all those affected by cancer end up with mental health ailments but it's important to take stock and check in with yourself to ask the question, 'Are you really ok?' And if you are not, then that is ok, too. The key is to acknowledge, accept and find the help that you need in whatever shape or form.

I didn't take stock of my mental health early on, from the panic attacks that initially ensued to the anxiety and claustrophobia that followed, to the PTSD after treatment ended. I only had the headspace to attempt to deal with it all fully after treatment ended. Despite thinking I didn't need a counsellor initially (clearly in the denial phase), I did, however, accept counselling five weeks after diagnosis as I cried inconsolably for four days straight after my stoma reversal, on the ward. Through these days on the ward, I journalled what had happened during the last five turbulent, life-altering weeks. It was like a ray of sunlight as Danni, my psychotherapist (who has already provided so much of her invaluable insight and expertise for this book), pulled the curtains back and sat with me. We started from the very beginning, and I read her my musings, and this was where our therapeutic relationship began and indeed continued for 18 months after.

I've learnt so much about mental health since cancer. I know I'm a GP and in fact a third of my workload involves management of mental health issues. However, I cannot express what a steep learning curve it has been. Within my job, mental health has been a passion of mine. I've not had mental health problems in the past. Now, experiencing some of what my patients face daily, my empathy gates have widened even more, which in itself can be a double-edged sword. The list below shows all the mental health states that I have experienced to different extremes through this past year, as do many individuals with life-changing illnesses or events. I've discussed some of these already, but I hope to talk about the others in more detail throughout this chapter.

- Anxiety
- Depression
- Loneliness
- Panic attacks
- Despair
- Low self-esteem
- Low self-confidence
- PTSD
- Panic attacks
- Grief reaction
- Phobias – worsening claustrophobia for me

What do I advise patients, and what have I learnt from my own experience and that of others? When it comes to your mental health, please put as much importance and time into managing this as you do into the physicality of treatment. It is such an investment for the long term – after all, cancer is a marathon, not a sprint. Towards the end of the chapter I'll talk about the toolbox that can help emotionally and mentally to support you during this time.

Anxiety

'People with anxiety don't have a train of thought. We have seven trains on four tracks, that narrowly avoid each other when paths cross. On top of this, all the conductors are screaming.'

Unknown

Depression and anxiety in cancer survivors/thrivers are common. Approximately 18–20 per cent of cancer survivors report symptoms of depression or anxiety within the first 12 months after treatment.

Poor recognition of anxiety and depression is associated with reduced quality of life and survival. So it is important to seek help, support and treatment for this.

Ensure you check with your oncologist if you do start antidepressants as some can react with chemotherapy agents.

Symptoms of anxiety can consist of physical and emotional symptoms:

Emotional symptoms of anxiety	Physical symptoms of anxiety
Uncontrolled worry	Tiredness
Inability to cope or feeling overwhelmed	Palpitations
Trouble concentrating, focusing thoughts or solving problems	Breathlessness
Irritability	Trembling
Sense of dread or impending doom	Excessive sweating
Constantly 'on edge'	Gut symptoms: nausea or stomach ache, bloating, constipation, diarrhoea
Restlessness	Pins and needles
	Dizziness
	Muscle aches and tension
	Dry mouth
	Headache
	Insomnia

Anxiety was a big part of my 'cancer experience'. It crept up on me silently soon after diagnosis, without me even realizing. I was so determined to stay in control, however, it gradually started at night, in the form of panic attacks, and the physical symptoms were more prominent as I managed to suppress the emotional state of my mind. As time went on, it manifested as worrying incessantly about things I knew I couldn't change. Situations, people, uncertainty. It stopped me from working early on after diagnosis. During chemotherapy I experienced anxiety daily, and at times it was paralyzing. I would at times struggle to get out and see people, go back on the school run and integrate back into society away from my sick bed. Yet, I still tried to go out with a smile attached to my face each day, trying to mask what I truly felt underneath.

Anxiety is a really challenging condition and one that I tried to manage through counselling, exercise (when I felt well enough) and, eventually, CBT. I cogitated about medication for a long time, especially after treatment ended, but never made the move. Maybe it would have helped, but I was in a place where I was tired of taking drugs and being reminded that cancer had left yet another gift.

It is important to seek help if:

- You are worrying most days or uncontrollably
- Worrying affects your daily life, usual activities and relationships
- Worrying impacts your mood or you are constantly upset

See your doctor for further treatment and advice including lifestyle- or therapy-based approaches, and medication.

Panic attacks

'I lied when I said I was busy.

I was busy but not in a way most people understand.

I was busy taking deeper breaths.

I was busy silencing irrational thoughts.

I was busy calming a racing heart.

I was busy trying to tell myself I was ok.

Sometimes this is my busy,

And I will not apologize for it.'

Unknown

Up to one-third of people will experience a panic attack at some point in their life. Factors that may increase the risk of developing panic attacks include:

- Family history of panic attacks or panic disorder.
- Major life stress, such as death or serious illness of a loved one.
- Trauma.

February 2020

It's 2 a.m. I can't breathe. I can't sleep. I think it's panic. Some PTSD? I'm going back to hospital in less than six hours.

For spinal injections.

We are flying away for my belated 40th, and I don't think I could manage the flying or travel we were planning right now with the sciatica how it is. TENS machine has been on full whack all week. The pain specialist thinks the sciatica is probably caused by lots of factors including cancer, chemo, trauma – mental and physical – surgery and a weakened core, hypermobility that I have, and the high-intensity exercise when my body wasn't ready post treatment.

So I'm so over the moon that I have a chance of being pain free and enjoying a trip of a lifetime to South Africa with my family before it's scan time again.

To compound matters, I also got my next CT surveillance date scan through yesterday which I'm sure has added to it all. I was hoping it wouldn't arrive till I got back from holiday!

But it's all coming out at night and each night before bed this week, I've found it a little more difficult to breathe and it's a really unpleasant sensation, but I managed to control it. Tonight I can't get a grip on it. It's irrational, but scary all at the same time. Feels like someone has taken over my lungs, sitting on my chest and I can't take enough oxygen in. It makes me feel even more claustrophobic. And breathing exercises are making it worse. Distraction is helping and sitting up!

Sorry I'm writing this now in a bid to try get some sleep … if I write it down … it might help? I can but try.

A panic attack can take you by surprise, be extremely frightening for you, and for others watching. It can come on very quickly and for no apparent reason.

During a panic attack you can experience a rush of intense mental and physical symptoms, which can include:

- A racing heartbeat
- Feeling faint
- Sweating
- Nausea
- Chest pain
- Shortness of breath
- Trembling
- Hot flushes
- Chills
- Shaky limbs
- A choking sensation

- Dizziness
- Numbness or pins and needles
- Dry mouth
- Ringing in your ears
- A feeling of dread or a fear of dying
- A churning stomach
- A tingling in your fingers/lips

Tips: How to manage a panic attack

I'm often asked by patients how they could best help reduce that overwhelming feeling of pure panic that describes a panic attack. Here are my strategies:

- Recognize you're having a panic attack and remind yourself you will not come to harm with this.
- Keep telling yourself that nothing bad is going to happen, and this is anxiety related. Do not fight it.
- Repeat mantras such as 'This shall pass'.
- Close your eyes, focus on your breathing. Breathe your way through them – in through your nose SLOWLY and out through your mouth. Count to 4 or 5 with each breath.
- Try to continue what you are doing in the same situation, confronting what is going on.
- Focus on peaceful/relaxing images or focus on objects. Focus on your happy place.
- Muscle relaxation techniques. This involves tensing up and relaxing various muscles in turn. To do this, hold the tension for five seconds. Say 'Relax' as you release the muscle. Let the muscle relax for ten seconds before moving on to the next one.
- Use a grounding technique, such as 5–4–3–2–1 (see below).
- Tell someone and explain what you need, if anything – so they can support you when it happens.
- Know your triggers – for example, small spaces/crowds – so you can start to anticipate/manage and hopefully reduce the frequency of episodes.

To try to prevent them:

- Talk to a therapist or obtain self-help books for CBT (your doctor will have a list).
- Practise mindfulness, yoga or Pilates.
- Take regular exercise to reduce stress and improve your mental health.
- Learn different breathing techniques.

- Avoid sugary foods, drinks, caffeine and alcohol, which can make attacks worse.
- Try massage, aromatherapy, calming activities.

Speak to your doctor for advice and possibly the need for medication to help.

5-4-3-2-1 grounding technique

This is a great and simple technique to help pull you back down to earth. Before starting this exercise, take a few deep breaths in and out and then focus on your environment, to invite your body and mind back.

5 – Look for five things around you – look in close detail, pay attention to the colour, the texture, the shapes.
4 – Become aware of objects around you and their touch – the scarf on your neck, the floor beneath you, the cold metal spoon.
3 – What can you hear? The trees, the birds, the traffic, the mobile phone in the distance.
2 – Acknowledge the smells around you – perfume, flowers, the damp air, your own natural smell.
1 – Identify one thing you can taste – the lingering taste of toothpaste, a chocolate.

Repeat this technique as many times as it takes to help you feel back where you belong, and at peace.

Depression

Sadness is a normal response to a cancer diagnosis, with the psychological, emotional and physical life-changing burden it can bring. I often found the treatment itself could cause some of these symptoms and this is normal.

Depression may result from chronic stress that overwhelms a person's ability to adjust to changes in life, leading to the symptoms below. Rates of depression are thought to be three times higher in cancer patients, compared with the general population.

Symptoms may include:

- Feeling low in mood, sad or tearful most days
- No pleasure or joy in life with things you used to enjoy

- Low motivation
- Changes in sleeping, eating and concentration
- Thinking about self-harm or suicide.

Having a cancer diagnosis, it is normal to have these symptoms from time to time. You may also only experience some of them or they can vary; however, if these symptoms persist, it is important to see your doctor for advice, help and support.

Your doctor can assess what the issues are, give advice on lifestyle changes to help manage your mood, refer you for talking therapy or a psychiatrist if needed and talk to you about medication options.

If you have thoughts of self-harm or suicide, please contact your medical team or doctor straight away.

Suicidal thoughts

Studies show that patients with cancer are at an increased risk of suicidal thoughts and suicide, probably at least twice as likely. The contributing factors including psychological and physical issues can no doubt lead to a reduction in the quality of life. Those who are at an increased risk are similar to those in the general population: male, increased age, those who lack social support, or those with pre-existing mental health illness.

However, different cancers have different suicide rates. With regard to colorectal cancer, there was a greater risk if cancers were towards the end of the colon or in the rectum. Presumably this relates to the quality of life post surgery of the lower end of the bowel and the end result often being a stoma, or subsequent LARS. I was never suicidal, but I will admit to a couple of moments of fleeting thoughts of 'What is the point?' – but nothing more than that. This was often at my lowest, sickest point in chemo when the drugs had completely taken hold, and the days of darkness would seem to drag on. I'd be willing myself to the toilet, yet felt so awful I couldn't get there. There were times of hopelessness and times where I couldn't see the light. But thankfully the curtains would draw, and light shone once more.

Checking in on those going through cancer is so vital, not just at the beginning and through treatment but also after. Please, please do ask for help for yourself or loved one if you ever find yourself in this position.

Claustrophobia

A fear of closed spaces.

Much of the panic I experienced from diagnosis and through treatment was related to claustrophobia.

Having claustrophobia in a mild form pre-cancer, I used to avoid enclosed spaces. But this was exaggerated immensely with treatment. From scanners, to oxygen masks, to tight cubicles. I found it difficult in lifts and even toilet cubicles, worrying incessantly that I would get trapped or locked in.

The sensation of not getting enough oxygen to your lungs. Impending doom. The world closing in. I can't escape. I can't get out. A metaphor for how I felt with cancer. With the symptoms getting worse, I decided my claustrophobia would be a priority in terms of management.

Standard treatments include desensitization or self-exposure therapy. This means you are gradually exposed to the stimulus that causes the fear and panic. If you are unable to do this on your own a therapist can help via CBT methods. Trauma-based CBT and exposure therapy have definitely helped alleviate my own symptoms which are more manageable and probably back to their pre-cancer baseline levels.

May 2020

Exposure and not avoidance, I've learnt through CBT, is key. And with the pandemic in full swing when I started trauma-based CBT, face masks were a good starting point as I couldn't even bear wearing these initially. The extra stress and panic at work in addition to the day-to-day stress of working in the health service during a global pandemic, I find myself continuously trying to talk myself down that I can breathe and I'm ok.

This has been a little difficult to face up to in this pandemic if I'm honest. But an excellent exercise for exposure and hopefully desensitization with time.

Maybe after I've mastered surgical face masks for prolonged periods, I'll try getting in a cupboard or one of those tunnels in the park. Not sure I'm quite there yet. I'll stick with just being able to cope with a face mask for now and get into a scanner without falling apart. What I've realized is that I need to try to stop the pattern of avoidance and deal with this head on.

Post-traumatic stress disorder (PTSD)

'A trigger is the connection between the conscious mind and a buried painful memory.'

Unknown

As you can see from what we have discussed so far, the impact of cancer is so widespread, not just with the physical burden, but from the emotional and psychological load. This has been likened to trauma experienced in natural disasters and one shouldn't underestimate the trauma cancer can bring, through the various stages from the investigations, procedures, diagnosis and treatment.

PTSD is a mental health condition that occurs after a traumatic event. It is a response to trauma, as our brains were not built to handle levels of such stress. It was known as 'shell shock' in the past as it was often recognized in war veterans. However, it can occur in response to other traumatic health events such as cancer.

I had no idea I was suffering with this. Initially, I didn't see cancer as a trauma till the aftermath where I permanently felt on edge. Symptoms include:

- Flashbacks
- Nightmares
- Intrusive thoughts or images
- Avoidance of reminders of a traumatic event
- Intense distress with any reminders of the traumatic event or triggers
- Insomnia/difficulty sleeping
- Anxiety
- Changes in mood or thinking
- People may experience loneliness, guilt and irritability with this as well.
- Avoidance of feelings and memories.

I constantly felt the need to be busy, burning myself out with absolute exhaustion. I would occasionally have nightmares about cancer, have panic attacks at night and became a complete insomniac. I would struggle with the daily triggers at work, and the loneliness and guilt would eat me whole some days. I think my husband would vouch for my irritability too! I felt a numbness at times and often talked about my cancer experience with my psychotherapist in a medical and detached way, as if I was watching from the outside-in.

Management of PTSD

Speak to your doctor if you think you might be experiencing PTSD. They may suggest any of the following:

- A 'wait and see' approach – do the symptoms improve with time or worsen without treatment?
- Antidepressants – paroxetine or sertraline
- Psychological therapies – such as EMDR (eye movement desensitization and reprocessing) or trauma-focused CBT.

What I'd like to highlight here is that, although trauma may change us permanently, healing from trauma is possible and we will talk about post-traumatic growth in Chapter 19.

How can we help manage our emotional and mental wellbeing?

'Our life is shaped by our mind, for we become what we think. When the mind is pure, joy follows like a shadow that never leaves.'

Buddha

I often say to those of my patients who are hoping for a quick fix and a magic pill that this indeed might help improve things, but it is rarely the solution long term. Unfortunately, like most DIY jobs, it is a multi-pronged approach, using a variety of tools, some of which you may prefer to use more than others. Like completing any home improvement tasks, it can be hard to get going, the motivation may be lacking and, when your mental health is suffering, trying to make positive changes can seem impossible. Having a toolbox of tricks to help manage our mental wellbeing in combination with any additional therapy or medication that we may need can really help, as well as aiding recovery.

My tool box: Tips and tricks I learnt along the way

Everyone needs a toolbox to help keep check of their emotional and mental wellbeing. Some tools are needed daily, some less frequently. Either way, you can choose what helps you. You may have other tools that you may utilize in addition to these. Suggestions include:

- Self-care (see Chapter 11) and compassion
- Eat well
- Sleep routine and sleep hygiene
- Talk, talk and talk
- Exercise
- Journalling, writing, gratitude journal
- Life cleanse
- Mindfulness
- Breath work
- Support groups
- Counselling
- Therapy

Compassion

'If compassion doesn't include yourself, it is incomplete.'

Buddha

Compassion.

Something I think I give out quite freely.

Something I have little of for myself.

Consider self-compassion a power tool that generates an understanding of ourselves and the way we feel, without judgement, rather than ignoring our pain or being self-critical. It's taking that moment to say, 'I'm not ok right now, but I'm doing my best and that will be enough.'

Self-compassion is consistently found to be related to better psychological outcomes. Yet the barrage of emotions attached to cancer can interfere with the simple process of being kind to ourselves. Guilt is a classic example: hindering our innate ability to treat ourselves as we would a loved one. Studies also show that those with cancer who instigate self-compassion throughout their cancer experience might reduce symptoms of anxiety, depression and fatigue, coupled with having a better quality of life.

I've learnt a huge amount about self-compassion, and therapy has taught me to be kinder to my body and myself. To ease the pressure from myself. I learnt to schedule rest into my weeks, and listened to my body when it came to exercising – without the baggage of emotions attached to doing so. This was always a marathon so to keep on running, even when my fuel cylinders were running empty, was foolhardy.

The model below has really helped me focus on elements of compassion which I hope you will find useful too.

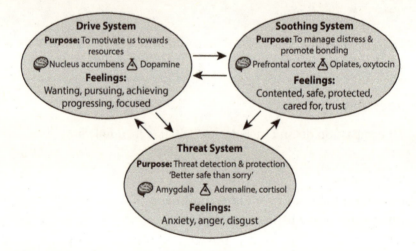

Figure 15.1

Compassion model – compassion-focused therapy (CFT)

CFT highlights the importance of compassion in interactions with yourself and the world. This is often used for trauma but can be used for other conditions too. Therapy sessions using this model aim to bring the three emotional systems into balance and promote healing. I found it extremely useful when things were getting too much, giving me some control to consider which system was dominating, and how I counteract this using other systems. The 'Soothing' system included many of the tools I will talk about below.

Let's take exercise, for example – it was my 'drive' to regain fitness and strength, and it also 'soothed' me in terms of helping my mental health, but it became a threat when I over-exercised, which exhausted me, and impacted my ability to parent and to work, leaving me needing more rest which I then didn't have time for. It highlighted the need to pull back. A similar interaction occurred when it came to my return to work – I had a drive to go back to feeling fulfilled, and have a sense of purpose, but it drained me and triggered me, so in turn also became a threat. As a result, I found I needed more things to 'soothe' me and counteract the balance.

Nutrition – eating well will also nourish your mind

The relationship between our mental health and our diet is complex. However, we know there is a link between your sense of wellbeing and your diet. Investing some time and looking at small changes in your diet may have significant benefits for the way you feel. See the 'Eatwell Plate' at https://assets.publishing.service.gov.uk/government/uploads/system/uploads/attachment_data/file/528193/Eatwell_guide_colour.pdf to show how an ideal meal should be divided in terms of nutrients.

Tips: Eating and drinking well

- Ensure you are drinking at least six to eight glasses of water or squash a day (this does not include tea or coffee). Mild dehydration can affect energy levels, your mood and ability to concentrate and be productive.
- Ensure you eat regular meals to stop blood sugar dips, which can make you feel like you're flagging or 'hangry' (irritable).
- Try to eat at least five portions of fruit and veg a day and include wholegrain for vital vitamins, minerals and fibre. Getting constipated can make you feel sluggish too, so try to avoid this.
- Include protein with every meal. It contains an amino acid that your brain uses to help regulate your mood.
- Ensure you are eating the healthy fats found in olive oil, seeds, nuts, oily dishes such as salmon, avocado and eggs. Your brain needs these fats to stay well. Avoid trans fats (or saturated fats) – often found in processed or packaged foods – as they can have a negative impact on not only your mood, but also your heart.

- Much has been discussed about the gut – brain axis and how your gut health can influence your mental health. We know that stress can impact your gut, causing it to speed up – resulting in diarrhoea – or to slow down, causing constipation. It is important to look after your gut microbiome with prebiotic and probiotic foods (see Appendix).
- Limit your caffeine as this can impact mood: it can cause irritability and insomnia, or increase anxiety. Caffeine is found in coffee, tea, cola, energy drinks and chocolate.

Sleep hygiene and sleep routine

For more on the restorative power of sleep, see Appendix.

Communication – talk, talk and talk

Cancer conjures up strong, pervasive emotions. Finding the ability to talk about them can reduce anxiety, can provide a relief from the burden as well as helping you feel seen and heard, facilitating the process of letting go. It can help make sense of what is going on around you by transcribing your thoughts into words.

I'm a big fan of talking. Had you guessed? No one can help, or no one knows to help, even those nearest and dearest, unless you ask or actually spell out how you are feeling. Who you choose to talk to is personal – someone who will listen to you without judgement is key – a partner, family member, friend, doctor, therapist. Opening up to those around you can also help them feel involved and valued.

Sometimes it is easier said than done, I know. It may help to speak to someone you don't know – in both the UK and beyond, charities like Macmillan have a support line, or you may find an online community or support group more helpful.

Exercise – release those endorphins

I've already talked at length about exercise in Chapter 11. When it comes to mental health benefits, exercise releases feel-good hormones which can also reduce pain, namely serotonin, endorphins and dopamine. Exercise boosts self-confidence and self-esteem, making us feel better about ourselves. It also boosts energy levels in the day, facilitates sleep at night, and is a stress reliever, reducing symptoms of anxiety and depression. It has been shown in studies that walking for an hour or running for 15 minutes can reduce your risk of depression by 26 per cent, and maintaining an exercise schedule can help prevent you from relapsing. It really is a powerful medicine for mental health, let alone the other health benefits, and if there is one thing I ask patients to do, this is high up in the list of self-help measures.

Journalling

'Fill your paper with the breathings of your heart.'

William Wordsworth

Writing a journal daily if you choose to can help focus the mind on your accomplishments, allow you to express your thoughts and feelings, as well as process what is going on. It can be used to express what you are grateful for and delve into thoughtful enquiry as to where you hope tomorrow may take you. This can intensify the pleasure of your experience each and every day. Some studies show that people who journal regularly see benefits to their physical well being, too.

I'll be completely honest, these are all things I have taken up since cancer. I wrote diaries when I was a child and later on holidays, but this was the first time in a long time.

Journalling for me became a crutch, something I didn't necessarily write daily but something that gave me a definite outlet and allowed the emotions to pour out. My husband would often describe my ramblings unpoetically as 'vomit on a page' as some days it felt I needed to purge myself clear of all the thoughts on to the page in disorganized chaos. It didn't matter, they were my words carved out on a page and they made sense to me, and I'd revisit these musings, and try to make sense of it all. It started as a simple pen and paper exercise, and then I turned to writing in the notes section on my phone so it was always accessible. I would often sit and reflect on these emotions for a couple of days, before I 'released' my musings publicly on to social media as part of my blog and catharsis. I would read each and every comment in response to this, many of which were from people who could relate or offer empathy and support at that time, which allowed me to feel seen and heard. The final part of the process was reading these extracts out to my therapist in a bid to make sense of them all, working through the turmoil chapter by chapter. This was all part of a therapeutic process that had inadvertently and organically grown, allowing me to move onto the next chapter.

If you decide to write a journal (for whatever reason), remember you do not need to show it to anyone if you choose not to, but it can be quite a liberating experience if you do. No one is there to judge or take their red pen out, it just needs to flow. It can also sometimes trigger emotions, so be aware and ensure you are in your safe space with strategies to ground you. There is no need for perfection, as evidenced by my journal entries through this book. They are raw and unfiltered.

Ideas for writing prompts

- Write down your story.
- How did a cancer diagnosis make you feel?
- Tell me about treatment.
- What was the hardest part of your cancer experience?
- How has it affected relationships?
- What would you tell someone who was diagnosed with cancer?
- Write down your worries.
- What makes you happy?
- What would you tell your younger self?
- How has a cancer diagnosis changed you?
- I am grateful for …
- I feel proud that …
- What I fear most is …
- I am relieved …
- Today, I am feeling …
- I am inspired by …
- What positive gifts has cancer given you?
- What have you learnt from your experience of cancer – the good, the bad and the ugly?
- How do you see life, moving forwards?

All I can say is give it a try, I never knew that writing would become such an important tool in my journey.

Gratitude journal

In each day, there is always something to be thankful for.

Unknown

We all have the ability to cultivate gratitude. Some days, it may be easier to focus on what is not going well, but taking a few moments to think about what you have at that present moment, and what has gone well that day, can quickly shift perspective. We know that those who express their gratitude are more likely to be optimistic, show resilience in adversity, have lower stress and anxiety levels, and be able to focus in the present. They tend to have better self-esteem and are maybe more forgiving or generous, thinking about ways to 'pay it forward'. Gratitude can also improve and forge better relationships as you take the time to appreciate those around you, and it can reduce irritability. That's a lot in itself to be grateful for!

There is no right or wrong way to write a gratitude journal, but there is always something to be thankful for. Find a peaceful moment for ten minutes; a good start is writing down five things you are grateful for in the day. Be detailed and specific about the act, thing or person you are thankful for.

Below is an example of an entry I made.

December 2019

- I am so grateful for the network of friends we have locally, the husbands have taken G on a night out, that I know he needs. Some respite from our daily reality.
- I'm so grateful for the delicious chicken pie a kind friend brought round tonight. The children absolutely loved it, and it didn't upset my bowels.
- I'm grateful that my feet and hands aren't too sore from the chemotherapy at the minute.
- Whoever invented bed socks is a genius! The warmth, comfiness and protection against the cold – priceless.
- I am grateful to be able to get out of bed and walk downstairs, rather than just lying in bed all day, to change surroundings and venture around the block and feel the sunshine on my back.

Remember what you feel grateful for doesn't have to be big and bold, it can be the small things that maybe wouldn't even get a mention otherwise.

Life cleanse

'Not all storms come to disrupt your path, some come to clear your path.'

Unknown

You have entered a new normal, and life is tough enough post cancer. What better time to look at life and reassess aspects of your life that you may not now need or desire? Reassess relationships – remove or minimize the impact on, and interaction with, toxic people from your life. Surround yourself with radiators, not drainers. Designate a screen- and technology-free space or have a social media detox. Declutter. Set boundaries. Reassess your schedule day-to-day, or revisit your diet and exercise regime. Small changes can make huge differences to how you feel. Eliminating harmful materials and replacing them with more beneficial ones can bring a new positive energy to your life.

Mindfulness that suits you

'Mindfulness is a way of befriending ourselves, and our experience.'

Jon Kabat-Zinn

Mindfulness is the process of bringing our attention to experiences happening in the present moment, while recognizing and accepting our feelings through a non-judgemental lens.

It is about slowing down, consciously noticing everything around you and within yourself. How your body feels, your breath, tuning into your senses – the sights, sounds, smells, the tastes. It is most definitely the opposite of the daily grind which can involve rushing around and multitasking furiously.

Cancer is a stressful event and can leave us dwelling in the past, maybe living with regrets, or being fearful of the future. Learning to live in the moment and be present (using mindfulness as a tool) can help you move forward, calm your mind, help your concentration and focus, and reduce levels of stress not only for the person with cancer, but for the carers surrounding them. It can alleviate anxiety and soothe the soul as well as helping chronic pain patients and those who are depressed. Denying our feelings can be counter-productive and impact negatively on our mental and physical health but mindfulness can help with this, and facilitate acceptance of them.

We know that it reduces the stress hormones in the body, cortisol and adrenaline, which are responsible for the 'fight or flight' response. Mindfulness also helps with the release of feel-good neurotransmitters, endorphins.

What works for one person doesn't always work for others, and like any new skill, mastering this requires practice and perseverance. Reassuringly, practising mindfulness does get easier with time. It is preferable for whatever activity you choose (it can be a different activity each day), to be performed daily for the greatest benefit, even if that's just five minutes a day.

I'll admit to being absolutely useless at this initially and I had to actively make time for it; it also took time to find a mindfulness exercise that worked for me.

I struggled at first when I listened to apps like Headspace or Calm, which provide guided meditations and mindfulness exercises. My mind would flit from place to place, never engaging in the moment at the beginning. As time went on, it became easier, but I also realized that other 'mindful' activities suited my personality better.

I found cooking to be very mindful. Looking at each ingredient, smelling it, tasting it, savouring the moment. I also found yoga and Pilates were mindful activities, drawing awareness to my breath and how my body was feeling at individual moments. And I decided to have tennis lessons, where I had to concentrate so hard on what I was doing, I thought about nothing else but the contact of the ball with the racquet.

Simple things such as stopping what you're doing and taking a deep breath; noticing the sensation of the breath; putting your phone down; focusing on one task at a time; and finding the mindful moments each day can help get you started.

Mindful activities can help anyone of any age, and there is a wealth of information online covering things like:

- Mindful eating
- Mindful walking
- Mindful breathing
- Mindful bathing
- Mindful creativity
- Colouring

- Yoga or Pilates
- Forest bathing.

What should happen when you perform any of these activities is that your focus becomes more present, you become more body aware, you are able to release tension and let go, while reducing the stress response in the body.

If you would like further information about mindfulness, please see the Useful Resources section at the back of the book.

Breath work

> 'Breathing in,
> I calm my body.
> Breathing out,
> I smile.
> Dwelling in the present moment.
> The only moment.'

Thich Nhat Hanh

As we breathe in, the breath takes oxygen around our body to all the cells as the blood pressure and heart rate rise. As you breathe out, blood pressure and heart rate drop once more and your body relaxes. When the body is under physical or emotional stress, this can impact how we breathe.

Breath work is an empowering practice that can aid our wellbeing. People have been using breath work for thousands of years, but it is becoming increasingly more popular, and its roots originate in yoga practice. Breath work refers to any type of breathing technique or exercise where your breathing pattern is intentionally changed, in the hope of providing the benefits below. The beauty is that this can be done anywhere.

Benefits of breath work may include:

- Improved mental clarity
- Reduced stress and anxiety, and mood enhancing
- Helps process trauma, and a reduction in the symptoms of PTSD
- Lowers blood pressure and resting heart rate
- Strengthens the diaphragm (the dome-shaped muscles at the base of your lungs)
- More time spent in deep sleep

- Increased happiness
- Deeper spiritual connection
- Stimulates the lymphatic system
- Reduces pain
- Increased energy and stamina
- Improves digestion
- Helps support posture
- Can help improve immunity.

There are several simple breathing techniques you can try below, one at a time. As these are performed, listen to your body and observe how you feel:

4–7–8 breathing	Deep abdominal breathing (diaphragmatic breathing)
Inhale for four seconds.	
Hold for seven seconds.	Lie down with a hand on your chest and a hand on your belly.
Exhale for eight seconds.	Take a deep breath through your nose, for a count of four, slowly filling your chest (lungs) and your tummy.
	Hold your breath for two seconds.
	On the exhale, breathe out through pursed lips and feel your lungs completely empty out as your belly button draws towards your spine for a count of six
Box breathing	**Warrior breath**
Inhale for a count of five.	Inhale and exhale 21 times with no pause.
Hold for a count of five.	At the end, carry out the box breathing above 4–5 times.
Exhale for a count of five.	

Support groups

Use the resources around you. You might find support groups online, in person, through charities, hospitals or social media. This is not only for your cancer journey but also for your mental health. They have the expertise and knowledge and can help you feel more understood. I found them a huge source of education and a fount of knowledge.

Counselling

February 2019

It really helped to offload to my counsellor again this week. I've seen her once each cycle and often read her my journal entries. Her support has been invaluable as she listens and facilitates problem solving. At first I think I expected her to give me answers, and of course this is not her role. She helps me 'park' issues that don't need to be dealt with till after treatment (saving any emotional energy for treatment) and stops me cogitating over issues that have sometimes developed often from overthinking, sleep deprivation or the drugs!

She accepts me for who I am, and I feel she has already got me sussed out. There is never any judgement and it really is my safe space to say whatever I like, without hurting anyone's feelings. And no problem is ever too big or too small. It's helping me take control of my life (something I don't feel I have a handle on right now).

Right now, all I know is that this counselling is helping me get through treatment as best as I can. It's a bumpy ride, but I find it is essential for refuelling, so we can go the whole distance and more.

Clearly there are many benefits to counselling. Counselling can offer you a helping hand to work through problems in a non-judgemental way. What was really striking for me was to learn that my thoughts (which could become intrusive and very real) were not actually fact at all, and actually teasing apart the feelings around a thought can help restructure your narrative. Other benefits include helping to reduce anxiety and depression, as well as improving self-esteem and self-confidence. I feel that counselling through treatment prevented my mental health from plummeting any deeper into the abyss. It can help you move forwards and look at each problem more objectively, giving it more perspective.

I was extremely fortunate that counselling was offered to me from the charity-run holistic centre (the Fountain Centre) attached to the hospital in which I received treatment. Little did I know how much Danni my counsellor/psychotherapist would help, or become such a pivotal part of my treatment. She has become a dear friend and her input into this book as a psychotherapist has been indispensable, and will hopefully give you the specialist knowledge you need.

All four of us received counselling: myself, the children and my husband. It gave us guilt-free permission to just let it all out, in the knowledge that no one would feel upset by anything that was discussed. It became part of my treatment programme and rehabilitation. The days when things felt untenable, Danni helped me see that indeed they were possible.

Finding a therapist you connect with is so crucial, and don't be afraid to see someone else if the 'fit' is not right first off.

Ask your doctor or local cancer centre where you may find some cancer specific-led counselling available in your area, too.

Therapy

> 'Recovery is a process. It takes time. It takes patience. It takes everything you've got.'
>
> *Unknown*

There are many types of psychological therapies available out there. The type of therapy you require, really is dependent on so many factors and I wanted to highlight that the type of therapy you need somewhere down the line, may in fact change.

I want to tease out some of the gems that I learnt through therapy, share my experiences and divulge some of Danni's wisdom from her years of providing counselling services and therapy for cancer patients and their loved ones specifically. Even as a doctor, I was initially dubious about how I was going to move forward, and whether I even needed a therapist. How wrong could I have been?

CBT – cognitive behavioural therapy

January 2020

I used to cry daily, not so long ago.

The frequency has certainly lessened as the wounds are healing, and the scars form deep.

It doesn't take much to trigger off a dark moment, a smell, a work situation, a sensation, a time or place. Sometimes something totally out of the blue. I'm definitely learning to cope with this better. Although after I had my port scar injected with steroid in my chest, to lessen the keloid scar recently, together with gut issues after Christmas, I had a two-day deep dip where it all came crashing back. And I regularly have moments where I have flashbacks to last year, that bring tears to my eyes. I think I may be gaining some more control now.

Well sometimes anyway.

I have panic at times to things that would not have stressed me previously. For example, why am I even planning things after my next scan when I don't know my fate yet? Luckily, these are briefer and short lived and I continue to plan in hope.

237

I'm lucky to be surrounded by people, who keep me afloat. Also the development and recognition of my own coping mechanisms have helped no end.

Although not always sustainable, the incessant keeping BUSY and distracted! Which leads to exhaustion and then impacts mental health further.

I wonder when I will feel ever feel peace again.

CBT is a type of talking psychotherapy, which encourages you to explore the interaction between your thoughts which can elicit feelings or emotions leading to a behavioural change which in turn increases potentially negative thoughts. By changing one, you can potentially change the other, and interrupt the cycle. It aims to break down problems into smaller, more manageable chunks.

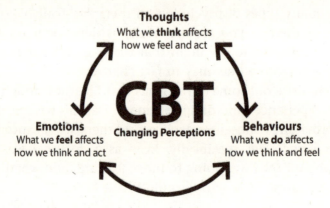

Figure 15.2 Cognitive behavioural therapy

It is goal orientated and aims to help identify specific and current problems and help address these, rather than focusing on what has happened in the past.

CBT can help a variety of conditions including depression, anxiety, PTSD, insomnia, phobias, obsessive-compulsive disorders and addiction. It can also be used for some people with physical conditions such as chronic pain.

You may have therapy on a one to one basis or as a group and there are often exercises or homework to complete at home. Together with your therapist you will identify the problem, thoughts, triggers and feelings, and set goals for the sessions ahead. One such exercise I did thoroughly engage with is the CFT model, discussed above, perhaps relevant and applicable to everyday non-cancer life as well.

EMDR and trauma-based CBT

'A note to anyone that needs to hear it: We don't 'get over' or 'move on' from our trauma. We are forced to make space for it. We carry it. We learn to live with it. And sometimes we thrive in spite of it.'

Unknown

EMDR (eye movement and desentization reprocessing) is a form of psychotherapy developed in the 1980s that was designed to alleviate anxiety and distress caused by traumatic events. Negative thoughts and feelings are thought to be a result of unprocessed memories. This technique alters the way traumatic memories are stored in the brain, making them more manageable. It uses side to side eye movements, sound or body tapping, along with talking therapy. The goal is to lessen the symptoms of PTSD by reprocessing, while staying anchored keeping one foot in the present and one in the past.

Trauma-based CBT

The other way to reprocess trauma is through trauma-based CBT. There are three phases of trauma-based CBT:

- **Phase 1: Stabilization.** This involves mapping the trauma, learning grounding techniques – methods to anchor yourself to the ground during a period of reliving trauma, as well as learning other techniques to help with the process to keep you 'safe'.
- **Phase 2: Narration and processing.** This is a technique to help trauma survivors make sense of their experience, while exposing themselves to reliving their story and painful memories: looking backwards through history, and using CBT techniques to aid processing.
- **Phase 3: Integration and consolidation.** This phase focuses on looking forwards into the future, consolidating the gains and techniques learnt in the previous two phases and applying these to everyday situations to develop a new and fulfilling life.

Below are passages written through time as I progressed through my course of CBT. They may be triggering for some, so please feel free to skip over till a time you would like to revisit this.

April 2020 – phase 1

Trauma-based CBT is in full swing and it's hard graft. There is no shadow of a doubt that it has rocked my mental wellbeing, and opening the can of worms seems never ending. There is part of me that still wants to believe that this didn't happen to me and staying in denial would be easier, and less destructive. But that is the purpose of this therapy. To allow you to reprocess the trauma in a 'healthier, more constructive' way. The timing is not great with everything going on (the global pandemic was in full swing), but it's all part of recovery and I just need to get on with it, as frankly I'm needed at work right now, and need to be firing on all cylinders.

Recognizing what drives me, what soothes me and what threats there are to my mood and how these can overlap is a great start, especially through these past few months.

I've had four sessions and had the last two weeks off which was a welcome break as I could just go into avoidance mode again and kid myself that I've dealt with cancer. Realistically I'm still in the process of dealing with it.

I still suffer from triggers. Many days I think I'm better and that I don't need therapy. Sure, on the face of it, it looks like I have it all under check. My reality of what's in my head is different at times. I feel a pressure to be positively grateful every day as I survived cancer. Yet I know it's ok not to be ok. But as I start the consult with my therapist, all the emotions come pouring out and flood gates open.

I find this therapy hard going, difficult and intrusive for many reasons.

Hard because I'm having to be truthful to myself, and not bury my head in the sand.

Hard because it's opening up old wounds, where all the debris hasn't been washed out.

Hard because I still don't truly accept I had cancer.

Hard because I couldn't cope with the loss of control to all aspects of my life during diagnosis, treatment and the aftermath. And I feel out of control again during therapy.

Listening back to what I was saying whilst reliving the first traumatic experience of my MRI, scans and diagnosis made me feel distinctly uncomfortable. I'm the doctor, NOT the patient. Surely. 'It shouldn't have been me.' 'Seeing my hospital name and number above the scanner doesn't feel right.' 'I was fit and healthy. I had no risk factors.' 'Every time I donned a hospital gown or was wheeled down the corridor, it felt so wrong…

And here was where the problem lay. **Doctors get cancer too.**

June 2020 – phase 2

Last week in CBT, I had to relive chemo. Deep breath. The sights, sounds, smells, tastes, sensations, everything about it. All in fine detail. It's amazing how much you can actually remember.

And I had a surprise cry initially at even this thought. She helped me ground myself (takes me back to a place of peace – for me this was a family holiday by the sea, far away in South Africa) and then I was guided through my story once more and started reprocessing. Healing the wounds. Raw wounds.

This week I had to read through my oncology letters. Can you believe I've not read one of them? Yet I read at least a dozen patient oncological letters a week at work for my patients. I would simply open it, and then leave it on my husband's desk to file in a mystery folder – I didn't even know the whereabouts till today. That's denial for sure.

So I started from the beginning. To allow my brain to acknowledge what happened. It was hard to read back. I felt sick. There were snippets of information in there that I was unaware of. Fascinating medical information too. All about my cancer, its whereabouts and the mischief that it played. Yet I thought, as a medic, I would have wanted to know more. I guess I felt I knew enough to know I just had to get on with treatment and plough through it. So at the time, I chose not to read them. As it made it real.

I was challenged by my therapist as I talked about loss of control so much, as to whether this was true fact. I know my voice was heard by my specialists, both surgical and oncology and my CNS, who were all key to my care too and driving it forwards. I may not have had control of treatment effects on my body or loss of control of my precious 'normal' life but my wishes were very much taken into consideration every step of the way. From taking a risk to go straight to surgery after balanced conversations with my surgeon and oncologist rather than opting for chemo-radiotherapy first (and its complications – and not everyone has a choice, I know), to early stoma reversal, to feeling completely toxic on chemo, and requesting help with this, too.

This very much challenged the loss of control issues that featured a lot during illness and treatment.

I think all in all, these processes are helping me come to terms with the car crash that occurred out of the blue. I think I can see that the avoidance behaviour in the long run would have led to further problems and potentially affected me at work, which in the long term is back where I would like to be.

July 2020 – phase 3

I've made it through phases 1 and 2. Phase 3 started today. So what does it involve?

Today, for the second time during therapy, I relived some of the traumatic aspects of diagnosis and treatment. The idea is to use the therapy we have been discussing to reprocess and try to form new adapted memories that are less traumatic.

We have been working on certain issues such as 'loss of control', 'denial and distraction', 'the strange and unnerving situation of being the patient and not a medic' and my acceptance of 'it's ok not to be ok' over the past few weeks. Today we drew together what I learnt to try to reprocess.

We tried to insert comments/thoughts that I would say to Anisha who was about to embark on diagnosis and treatment 20 months ago, in order to try to form these new adapted memories surrounding traumatic episodes.

So, bearing in mind that I accept that I did the best that I could at that time, what would I say now to me back then (and anyone else about to embark on a similar journey)?

1. It's ok to be frightened.
2. You can do this, and you will be ok.
3. Be kinder to yourself, more compassionate, less critical, less harsh.
4. Don't feel guilty, it's not your fault. Loved ones will still love you no matter what.
5. It's ok to change as a person and grow in a different direction, to change perspective on life (often for the better) and for relationships to change.
6. Allow yourself to go through the stages of grief … so eventually you can reach acceptance.
7. Distraction is ok short term but not long term. Long term, it is exhausting and you are not dealing with the issues at hand.
8. It's ok that you felt this was so foreign and strange. To be the patient and not the doctor. It is understandable and you've acknowledged that having knowledge has made it harder for you personally.
9. It's ok to lean on others and not be temporarily available to your loved ones. You are not failing, you haven't failed your children, your family, your husband, your friends … but in fact you succeeded in getting through treatment, with the best possible outcome for your stage of cancer, getting back to work, being a mum, being healthy and strong despite whatever post treatment threw at you physically or mentally.

It's been quite an eye opener with the exercises I have been doing with the therapist and I'm hoping as therapy comes to a close in a few weeks that the effort and engagement in this process will indeed help me moving forwards with life after cancer.

I successfully completed 12 arduous but enlightening sessions of trauma-based CBT. It was emotionally draining but I'm so glad I found a therapist I bonded with, and it very much helped many of the symptoms I was experiencing. I may not have forgotten but I'm definitely not living on a knife edge day to day anymore.

Four years on, I have compiled my own toolbox, and my awareness of my own mental health is finely tuned. I have a low threshold to pull tools out the bag when needed. Having insight into, and awareness of, how you are feeling is often half the battle.

I hope you will find your own toolbox to help you manage your emotional and mental wellbeing, and please seek professional help if your mood is deteriorating or symptoms are persistent.

I'll leave you with some self-affirmations I made in July 2019.

Know it's ok not to be ok.
Don't be ashamed.
You are not weak.
There should not be a stigma.
You are not alone.
Your feelings are valid.
And although it's hard to believe some days,
You are loved more than you know.

17

Relationships – living and loving after diagnosis

Relationships with your partner or loved one

I'd like to think that my husband and I have come through our collective experience a more tightly bonded couple, stronger than ever. And that is true, most of the time …

But getting to where we are today wasn't easy.

Cancer takes its toll on EVERYTHING, including relationships. You have to fight hard to stay on track, to not lose sight of what you're fighting for. There is a level of perseverance required similar to that needed to get through cancer treatment, especially during those interminable days where you feel you have nothing left to give and where the light at the end of the tunnel is no brighter than a distant dying star. Some relationships strengthen, some pre-existing cracks widen, and some relationship structures that were thought to have been built on the most firm of foundations simply crumble, inexorably, to dust.

Cancer is the roadworks that can create one-way traffic in a relationship, and it is important to address that imbalance as early as practically possible. After all, it is about getting your loved one through treatment too! Remember, it is not your carer who is the centre of attention, but without a shadow of a doubt they are the writer, director and producer of the show, the pivotal driving and caring force behind the patient, the unsung hero.

But with time, a dangerous pressure cooker of both guilt and resentment can build for patient and partner alike, and it is important to recognize this early, so that the valve can be released and steam vented.

And cancer changes you both as people. You try to find a way to reconnect, to be on the same page, perhaps even reading the same book! And to say it can be challenging would be an understatement.

And the rewiring needs to occur not only with each other but with friends and family too. Which takes time, hard work, and (as Elvis said) a little more conversation, possibly with a dash of therapy thrown in too.

G is my rock. He always will be. My cancer Buzz Lightyear – 'Through treatment and beyond!'

But how many people asked him how HE was doing? How HE was coping? How HE was feeling? During treatment, he was often the conduit for information about me, and with his specialist knowledge about the problem at hand, I think people's conversations with him were often more for their own reassurances about my welfare than for his. And this is probably true for most cancer patients, most of the concern is focused on the patient's wellbeing, as the person directly affected by the disease and its consequent treatment.

But I know that to him the small gestures and acts of kindness meant so much, and spoke volumes. Dropping off a beer with a food bundle, asking whether he fancied a gym session or a bike ride, or just asking him outright, 'How are you?' He certainly never asked for, nor expected, anything as recompense for his efforts, but the token gestures were more than payment enough.

And after a year of continuing to work full time with bowel cancer patients, be a fabulous carer and father and keep the house running, it is perhaps not surprising that the events of the year finally took their toll. And I lost my rock, albeit temporarily. And I crumbled too. It became too much for either of us to cope with, a mixture of emotions – exhaustion, anger, resentment, sadness and uncertainty ...

I recall a lovely elderly patient came to see me one week, telling me in depth how he was finding it so difficult to see his wife go through breast cancer treatment. How gruelling it was for her. He described it as torture to watch, and it took a toll on his mental health. He felt anxious, and helpless, and he fretted constantly about their future. He felt he had lost his wife in spirit, as she could do so little at the time. He had many a sleepless night filled with worry and dread, and above all he felt unassuageable guilt for eventually falling apart. He didn't know if he could live with the uncertainty. We had a very long consult.

Thankfully, I knew where to signpost him. On this occasion, it was to the local Macmillan Cancer Centre at the local hospital to see a counsellor there who specializes in counselling those afflicted by cancer or their loved ones. I also discussed the fact that everything he felt was normal as a carer, and told him that he was doing a fabulous job under very difficult circumstances. I encouraged him to confide in friends and family, but he was adamant he didn't want to burden them. His resilience was at an all-time low.

I think G would have had a very deep and meaningful chat with this patient, too. He'd also lost, albeit temporarily, the one person he could confide in. I simply didn't have the headspace or emotional resilience to help him come to terms with his own emotions at the time. I was still working through my own, which was extremely one sided, but as my counsellor said, I had to be able to paddle my own raft before I could take on any other passengers, and quite frankly, the raft was sinking in the rapids at that stage, so probably best he didn't try to climb aboard! And so, G courageously did reach out for himself, to seek help for our relationship and to help him move beyond what had been our 'annus horribilis'. He sought counselling at the same facility which had looked after both me and our children. Respecting each other's individual cancer experience, we have never spoken to each other in any depth about the conversations we had during our counselling sessions. But for him, it was a safe space where he could vent his frustrations, question the injustice, and learn to both voice and confront the 'dark thoughts' that began to pervade his waking hours.

And I'm so pleased to say that, by reaching out when he did, and getting the help he needed when he did, my rock came back.

Some relationships do emerge unscathed from under the cancer umbrella, but others falter. Often after cancer treatment has finished, some partners or carers find it difficult to understand why their partner is not back to normal, while others are unable to comprehend the anguish they still feel both physically and mentally in the aftermath of the cancer storm.

There are many things you can do that might help lessen the impact of cancer on relationships, and suggestions for working through them, from Danni, my psychotherapist:

- Talk, talk, talk. This can be difficult, so sometimes writing it down can help. Sometimes barriers can build up when communication lacks between parties, and outlining how you both feel is a start. Danni has observed through her work that the crevice between couples often widens, with a lack of communication, skirting around subjects and tiptoeing around the awkward topics. Danni can't stress enough to you, and to her clients, that you should be open and honest. Acknowledge the diagnosis and both of you share your fears. Recognize changes you have gone through physically, mentally and emotionally, and as a couple.
- Different values and different opinions may become more apparent when cancer enters your lives. It is important to listen, acknowledge, validate and respect this difference rather than feel that one person is exclusively right and the other wrong. This isn't always easy and may not sit right with you, but compromise is key.
- Sexual relationships can become strained, which can have an impact on a couple. I've written about this below.
- Emotional connection; as you transition back from patient to partner, a reconnection in this manner needs to occur. Think of ways to reconnect, something you enjoyed doing together in the past or something you would like to do together in the future.
- Be patient. It may be a long process to feel that things are back on track as you both learn that life doesn't automatically go back to normal. It will take time for the person who has cancer to recover, which in itself can be a lengthy process.
- Consider therapy – whether that be for yourself, your partner or as part of couples' therapy to aid any difficult conversations and break down any barriers.

Don't forget about the carers

Firstly, to all the carers out there, caring for someone with any condition, you are doing a phenomenal job during what must be one of the most challenging and loneliest of times. Please know that we would be totally adrift without you.

Your loved one may not be able to be the person that you need them to be, or be the support that you were accustomed to before cancer made its appearance, but don't be afraid to reach out. To friends, to family, and to your doctor.

Below I share a few tips for the carer and tips for those of you that know a carer and how you can best support them.

Tips for the carer	Tips to support a carer
Communication – be open and honest with those around you	Offer them an ear and actively listen. Check in and make sure they are ok – a text, email, voice mail or phone call. It will mean the world to them, I promise you
Look after yourself – eat well, exercise, sleep, take breaks and time for yourself, attend your own health appointments	Offer practical help, for example food shops, cooking, childcare, a night out, some respite from looking after their loved one
Remember your loved one may not be acting as they usually do, may be emotional, may say hurtful things. This isn't an excuse for them, but try to take a step back from the emotion and, as hard as it is, try not to take it personally	If you want to gift something to the family or patient, ask if there is anything they especially need
Support groups like Carers UK or Macmillan can offer support as well as practical advice, e.g. financial	
Seek help if you are struggling from your doctor or a counsellor/therapist	

Here's some advice from a close friend, who has found himself in the role of carer recently. All relationships are different, but these tips might help your relationship with the person you are caring for.

Tips: For carers

- Give yourselves the time and space to familiarize yourselves with the changes and the new roles as patient and carer.
- Keep communication channels open and ensure you talk regularly to circumvent issues building up. Ask what support the other needs and discuss ways of fulfilling this.
- Try to maintain some normality, structure and routine in your lives.

- Find the humour where you can. The days can be long. There were many times when we ended up laughing instead of crying in certain cancer-related situations. This can help alleviate some stress and after all, laughter is often the best medicine!
- Remember to schedule regular treats for yourself – date nights, takeaways, trips to the movies – whatever works for you, even if that might involve you running to the toilet every ten minutes in the early days (yes, that was indeed our first date night, trying to watch a film together!).
- Ensure the person being looked after remains in control, has a say in decisions affecting them, and can voice their opinion freely.
- Try to formulate ways that both parties can continue functioning as independently as possible.

If you are unsure how to get help, you can ask your cancer specialist nurse, Macmillan team, local cancer centre or your doctor for the support you may need as a carer.

Taking the taboo out of sex and cancer

My hope is that, after you read this section, you will feel less embarrassed to find a way to improve your sexual well being if it has been affected by cancer and its treatment, and if you do feel embarrassed, that you at least have some tools to help.

Cancer and cancer treatment can certainly impact sexual health and this is one of the concerns many cancer patients face in a number of different ways, physically and emotionally. Some treatments may have a bigger impact than others but every problem big or small is valid, and with survivors and thrivers living longer, relationship issues are becoming that much more important to address. Not only can this change in sexuality impact your quality of life negatively, it also impacts that of your partner.

Some people may be fortunate and feel no change to their sexual function, and want to keep having sex. This is fine, if it is safe to do so. There may be some circumstances where your oncology team may want you to avoid sexual intercourse.

The table below outlines the different reasons why sex lives can change for patients with cancer.

249

Men	Women
Side effects of treatment – pain, nausea, fatigue, vomiting	Side effects of treatment – pain, nausea, fatigue, vomiting
Emotional – anxiety or depression	Emotional – anxiety or depression
Lowered libido	Lowered libido
Altered body image/self-image	Altered body image/self-image
Changes in orgasm intensity	Changes in orgasm intensity
Erectile disorder	Menopausal symptoms, such as vulvovaginal dryness, hot flushes, and painful intercourse
	Changes in sexual sensitivity, such as nipple sensitivity

Who can I talk to?

It is not uncommon for cancer treatment to overshadow these sorts of problems and all too often, patients may feel anxious or embarrassed to talk about sexual health concerns.

As well as talking to your partner, when it comes to looking for help if your sex life is affected, it's important that you raise this with a health professional that you feel comfortable with. Remember before I talked about how to approach and prepare for a consultation, talking about a topic you may feel uncomfortable or embarrassed about? Use the same principles and tools given there, when you are working up to talking about this with your health professional. Remember to outline the issue clearly, then discuss your ideas, your concerns and your expectations.

> For example, sex is painful (*issue*), I think this is because I have vaginal dryness (*idea*), and it's affecting my relationship and causing distress (*concerns*). Can you help me as I would like to continue having sex (*expectation*)?

Writing your thoughts down and showing your doctor may make it easier for you to explain, too.

Tips: How to, metaphorically, get back on the horse

- Communicate with your partner and discuss each other's needs.
- If at first you don't succeed … keep trying and keep things light-hearted, be patient: it doesn't always happen first time.
- Maintenance sex – a concept where sex is almost diary-entried in, maybe trying a time of day to have sex when you feel least fatigued. It may seem unromantic but can help break periods of abstinence.
- If you tire during sex, rest – take a break.
- If you are really struggling with symptoms that make sexual relationships difficult, please speak to your healthcare professional, so you can hopefully come up with a plan for support.
- Intimacy is not just about sex. The brain is an important sex organ and the skin is the largest sex organ – the possibilities are limitless:
  - touching and stroking
  - kissing
  - massaging
  - talking
  - holding hands.

You have the right to the best quality of life possible with the treatment that has been undertaken. So please remember, your sexual health matters.

Intimate relationships with a stoma

It is not unusual to lose your desire for sexual intimacy after abdominal surgery. Re-establishing intimacy after having a stoma is a two-way process, which will require a period of adjustment and time. Naturally, the person who has the stoma may feel anxious and worried. There may be fears of rejection, feelings of self-consciousness and it is possible their self-esteem and body confidence may have changed. The partner, on the other hand, may feel worried about hurting the person with a stoma or even dislodging it. Communication and patience between the two individuals is key.

For other people with abdominal ostomies, sexual function may or may not change. Women could sometimes have pain during sex (use lubrication, avoid deep penetration or change position). Men may have trouble getting and keeping an erection. These effects are not usually long lasting.

What happens if you meet someone new, who has not been through the surgery and the process with you?

If a relationship is becoming serious, it is definitely worth discussing your stoma before the relationship becomes physical, to avoid any awkward surprises later on. Sometimes you can rehearse or write down what you want to say if that is easier, discussing why you needed the stoma in the first place.

If their reaction is such that they do not want to continue the relationship, there are a few things to remember. Firstly, people without stomas are rejected for all sorts of reasons and secondly, if they have a problem with you having a stoma, the relationship was probably not going to work from the outset.

I need to emphasize that people with stomas can have fulfilled relationships and sex lives.

Tips: Intimacy when you have a stoma

- Empty the stoma bag beforehand.
- Change positions if the stoma is in the way.
- Wear open panties, intimacy wraps, or a short slip or nightie. Men may consider wearing a cummerbund (wide support band) to secure and conceal the bag or use a pouch covering.

Do speak to your stoma care nurse if problems are ongoing.

Friendships – make or break?

Be prepared.

Some bonds will become stronger and unbreakable. Others will fall by the wayside.

The most important piece of advice I can give is, find your tribe. Do not waste time or energy on negative relationships (let them go – you have no surplus headspace for this right now), but invest yourself in those which allow you to mutually flourish.

You may find that some people stop spending so much time with you and others in fact invest more time with you. You may even make more friends (such as the cancer community I formed and bonded with online). Most of these changes will, hopefully, be positive ones.

We touched on people's reactions, and friends and their behaviours, and how you can help support your friend in Chapter 4. Again, as I always say, keep talking, and be honest, this time with your friends. They are not mind readers and may have misconceptions about what you may need. For example, if it feels like your friend is avoiding you, they may not know what to say, or think you are too ill to chat and are therefore letting you rest, or they may be worried about saying the wrong thing, or feel uncomfortable talking about cancer. They may think you're not up to visitors or feel guilty that you have cancer and they are still having fun, so don't want to upset you.

I felt upset sometimes when the world carried on around me, and there were times I could feel forgotten about, contrary to what anyone would say, so here are a few hints to help you feel connected and maintain relationships.

Tips: Maintaining relationships

- Ask friends to keep inviting you to things, with the proviso that you will go if you feel well enough.
- Ask them to keep calling or texting, even if you don't feel like talking. It makes you feel more seen and less alone, or forgotten about.
- If you want to talk about cancer, but you're not looking for solutions, ask them just to listen.
- If you would like visitors at home, or you are able to have them in hospital, let them know what to expect, your appearance may have changed.
- Remember they will be dealing with their own emotions too, but ask them to lean on others for the foreseeable future, until you're at a point where you can be leant on once again.

Ultimately friendships should be a source of unconditional support, love and fun, being there for you through the ups, downs and everything in-between.

When they bring gifts

Many people want to bring gifts. At one point shortly after diagnosis, I walked into my kitchen and remarked, 'Who's died? It looks like a funeral parlour in here!' I walked straight back out and my husband was left speechless, and probably not amused by my dark humour.

Don't get me wrong, I loved the flowers, but I never had the head-space or energy to clear them up, my friends would end up tidying or arranging them. Of course I missed the flowers when they stopped coming, and now and then, I gift them to myself as an act of self-love!

Most people undergoing cancer would say that the biggest (and best) gift people could give is time, even if that's over the phone. There is, however, a whole host of gift suggestions (which I collated from the cancer community), and what to offer is a question I commonly get asked by friends.

There were the practical gifts which were so thoughtful and much needed – gloves, scarves (big ones double up as blankets), hats, snacks, paraben-free toiletries including face creams, potions for dry skin, soft toothbrush, pyjamas, fluffy or cashmere socks, bed socks, silk pillow case for chemo, hot water bottle or wheat bag, a book with affirmations, water bottle, headphones, sweets or chocolate for chemo, a journal, a colouring book, vouchers for food delivery such as Cook, and so on.

And then the 'me before cancer' gifts – I also still loved receiving things that were a reminder of me and not cancer-related. Sparkles, jewellery, lipstick and sparkly eye shadow were some of my favourites. Another idea is buying them a treat – a massage, or clubbing together for a trip away.

Don't forget you can also gift yourself, for getting through different stages – my first present to myself was an electric blanket and I never looked back. After that, it was lots of sequins and impractical gifts to myself in the hope that I'd be able to don them somewhere special soon or, failing that, just wear them to chemo!

There are some great websites offering cancer-friendly gifts, cosmetics etc. (see Useful Resources).

The impact on children

For a moment, I also want to consider the impact of cancer on children. It's one thing having to stare cancer in the face, it's another when this spills over to your family, and to your children – it can be punishing on so many levels.

'Are you going to die soon Mummy?'

These are words that no young child should have to even think about.

The children never asked me this question directly when I was in treatment. I felt the main upset for them was the impact of treatment on me, which affected their lives through my resultant lack of presence in it.

While on holiday after treatment finished, my son (a year older) opened up after he watched me conquering my demons and fears, crawling through a tunnel in a playground as part of exposure desensitization therapy, to overcome the claustrophobia I'd developed from all the scans I had been through. As I emerged from the playground tunnel, a little shaky, K immediately held my hand tightly as we spoke about fears openly, and how we can try to overcome them. I asked him what he was scared of. After telling me in great depth about his fear of heights, he said the following:

K: 'Mummy, my teacher asked me why I was quiet sometimes and what I was frightened of when I was at school when you were ill. And I just sat and didn't say anything.'
PAUSE
Me: 'So what were you frightened of?'
K: 'That you were going to die.

I was not ready to hear that.

I spoke to the therapist at the time about this conversation and the guilt that ensued, my children having already seen me upset and distressed after embarking on the playground tunnel. But in true therapist-style, she pointed out the positives, for which I was utterly grateful. She told me the children saw my strength and determination to overcome my fears, that what they had just witnessed displayed my vulnerability (which humanized me), but it also allowed my son a chance to say the very thing that we had all at some point feared, which none of us at any point had dared to verbalize out loud.

What was truly remarkable was the children's resilience, and what was refreshing was their brutal honesty.

It was also their observations that touched me the most.

September 2019

My seven-year-old daughter snuggled up to me last night as I lay in bed feeling rough and spontaneously remarked, 'I think you are brave Mummy.' I asked her why. This is what she told me.

She thought I was brave for having another blood test and scan. And was also disappointed to find out why I would keep needing them for a little while, after she asked me directly why I still needed tests.

She told me, I was:

Brave for having another colonoscopy.

Brave for having my chemo daily and not making a fuss. Even when it made me feel poorly.

Brave for going into hospital on my own, and staying there for days at a time.

Brave for having a stoma although temporary.

Brave for working hard to get better, when it didn't always look easy.

And, finally, brave for having, in her words, 'fought' cancer.

Children never cease to amaze me. Their minds are constantly processing. I don't think I was brave. I did what needed to be done. And actually there are far braver people out there tolerating greater hardships and ill health. But in her world, I'm glad she thinks I was.

I'm also glad she doesn't remember me throwing my toys out of the pram on occasions.

And just so the children know ... the real brave ones are them! They are brave for so many reasons, I can't even begin to list all of them. For enduring a tough time, losing their mummy for a period of time, watching the emotional and physical rollercoaster of this past year and embracing the new normal we try to live fearlessly.

You know something?

You are braver than you know.

My daughter also wrote this piece for the book, her take on what she remembers of the impact of cancer when she was six years old. She is now ten.

My name is Shani, and I am ten years old. When my parents first told me my mum had been diagnosed with bowel cancer I was only six. At first, I didn't really understand what all the fuss was about because I was still quite young. The first few weeks I struggled to concentrate in school as I knew my mum was in hospital. Slowly, I started to understand what everything was about. The cancer. The surgery and chemotherapy, which would take the cancer cells away. Friends and family would come to our house to give food, love, and support. My uncles, Nanna, Nan and Grandad and lots of our friends supported us and helped us all the way through this unusual adventure. After a few weeks my mum started taking a large amount of pills every morning. I would sometimes feel upset seeing my mum sick in her room. We went to lots of people's houses and many people helped us. At school I would talk to a teacher to help me talk about my different emotions out loud. There were days where I felt strong and secure but there were other days where I felt lonely and scared. The thing I was most grateful for was all the support my family and I had. After four years, today I am so grateful for everyone but mostly that my mum is here today.

And here is my son's recollection (he's now 11).

Hi, my name is Kiran and at the time my mum had cancer, I was 7. It was a frightening experience and when we found out, we knew that there would be hard times ahead, but I'm pleased to say my mum has fought through the bad times, and the light has returned.

What helped me through it was the Fountain Centre, where we could go and see our counsellor, Julie. She was very kind, and gave us top tips how to get through the hard times. Everyone from our family and friend groups would help by making food, coming round for a chat, and helping pick us up from clubs and activities. It was nice and comforting to know that there were people looking out for our family. My dad was very busy all the time but still managed to fit in helping us and my mum, as well as working very hard. My friends were very supportive as often, going into school, I would be upset.

My mum tried her hardest to go out with us and even go on holiday – she managed but needed help along the way. When we had to change the poo bag [stoma], I would always run away, as it scared me, seeing my mum's inner body. Most of the time, though, she tried to stay in bed but she just couldn't sit still some days.

I would help as much as I could by taking food for her or bringing up water. We had to let her rest so my sister and I would make dens, read books and make art and crafts. Thankfully, lots has changed. MY MUM IS FREE FROM CANCER! It is much better, and my mum is feeling better than ever. All my friends have seen this book, seen her on TV, and she is a real life legend. I love my mum, and now I really know how much of a hero she is.

What can you do to help minimize the impact on children?

29 January 2019: cycle 3 – the drug-free week

Since Monday, I've been getting myself organized for the final round of chemo and to my children's delight (and mine), being mum again and fulfilling some of my motherly duties! As they start to worry about chemo starting again, I've made photo books for them to hopefully help see them through this next and final cycle, packed with memories and good times we have shared. We have also booked for them to see a counsellor next week and G thankfully has carer's leave for the 'bad' week, which will provide some normality and continuity that they are so desperately seeking now. They even had their first after school playdate at our house since my op, with a little help from a dear friend S (it's been three months since we've had children round to play here). This was a huge deal for the children, but actually also for me as well. I felt I was fulfilling part of my motherly role once more. The children's excitement was palpable and my heart just melted!

- Be honest, avoid hiding things if possible. Keep conversation channels open, as mentioned before, and be led by your child.
- Try to keep as much routine and normality as possible. Encourage your children to continue having fun and doing the things they enjoy without guilt.
- Give them time and space to process and try to work things out for themselves.
- If you have extended family or friends locally, call on them to help, they can be an invaluable source of support.
- Allow them to vent their emotions. My husband reassures me regularly that I haven't scarred my children for life but actually, if anything, this has shown them that in the face of adversity, you can fully turn things around and even go on to achieve great things. One of the key things is to allow your children an open space for them to set free any emotions that may be weighing them down. Long term this will be beneficial for their mental health too.
- Beware of behaviour changes – uncharacteristic behaviour changes could signify stress, distress, upset, anger and confusion they may be experiencing but having difficulty expressing or communicating. Although it's important to maintain boundaries, it's also important to be aware that behaviour may be out of character due to the emotions they are experiencing, and giving them that outlet with some of the tools below may help.
- Give the child or teen the tools to manage their emotions, and to vent their feelings:
  o Give your child a worry monster or worry box. My children were given these and found them incredibly useful – the furry teddy monster has a zip over its mouth and children can write their worries on strips of paper, post them through its mouth, and zip it back up. Every so often when the children were ready, we would unleash all the worries and go through them one by one with the children.
  o Encourage journalling (for an older child or teen).
  o Talk to them in the car or while doing something so they don't have to have eye contact with you. I sometimes found we had the most meaningful and open conversations during this time.

- o Let them know it's ok for them to speak to anyone they trust in school or a close friend or family, they don't have to talk to you.
- o Be creative: use art as therapy – painting, drawing, doodling, or use Play-Doh.
- o Ask someone the children know well and trust (extended family, friend) to keep a watchful eye on how they are coping. If you've let the children know they can talk about your diagnosis and treatment, they may open up and talk about their feelings or concerns, without the fear of upsetting you.
- o Speak to their school – they may be able to appoint a counsellor or an ELSA (emotional learning support assistant).
- o Books – a list of useful books can be found on the Fountain Centre website (see Useful Resources).
- o Have 'special time' when treatment allows.
- Show them how you feel – it's ok for them to see you upset and then cheer up. It means they have permission to do so.
- Play therapy or counsellors depending on their age (I'll never forget when K had to name the things that made him happy – pizza and football, and things that made him sad – couscous and cancer … yes couscous, according to seven-year-old K, was as bad as cancer!).
- Support groups – in the UK, you can find your nearest support group related to cancer for any service using the Cancer Care Map (see Useful Resources).
- Congratulate yourself, you are navigating a code red situation with no instruction booklet and you are still showing up each day. You may not be able to be there physically or mentally at times, but you will in your own way do what you need to do to ensure your children know they are loved. Do what you can do.

It is normal to feel parental guilt when faced with a cancer diagnosis. If I think about it for any length of time, the cancer guilt engulfs and consumes me. So, most days, I try to remember how this experience has enriched my children's lives and they have had life experiences as a result – both positively monumental and also earth shattering, all of which will no doubt add to their lives' tapestry.

The guilt I feel for the time I missed out with them during treatment and in recovery has been turned on its head, as our time is now crammed with making memory-type experiences which can be exhilaratingly exhausting.

We talk about cancer and death openly, about body parts, about health concerns, worries and issues that concern them. I'd like to think our children have the emotional intelligence to show others compassion and kindness when faced with hardships, and they were forced to become relatively independent at a young age, getting involved with household chores, cooking and generally mucking in. I hope my experience has sculpted them into well-rounded, empathetic, kind and considerate individuals, and I can only hope that my illness has had no long-lasting effects for them in the future.

I can't change the days I lost with my children, but what I can do is try my best to be there for them today, and show them how to live life to the full.

As the late Dame Deborah James said, 'Have no regrets.' I'd suggest you do exactly the same where you can – live for the moment, make memories with your friends and family that you can all hold on to through the good and the bad times, and nurture all the wonderful and positive relationships in your life.

18

Returning to work

Not everyone is able to return to work or to the job that they were performing prior to cancer due to treatment, side effects or disability. However, for those who find themselves returning to work, it's a huge step and a monumental milestone in the recovery process. It takes pure courage, so congratulations getting to this point.

Working With Cancer (see Useful Resources) is a self-funded social enterprise in the UK which helps employees, employers and the self-employed, and carers, to manage cancer and work. They carried out a survey and found that 80 per cent of cancer patients felt it was important to continue working, and 47 per cent had to give up their work and change roles as a result of their diagnosis. It was reported that unfortunately, one third of patients had negative experiences on their return to work too.

Anyone who has followed me on social media for a while knows this – that returning to work as a doctor has not been easy for me. At the time, I felt it was the right thing to do. I needed distraction, I wanted to feel purpose, but admittedly I felt pushed back to work with a degree of self-inflicted guilt, as my senior partner had been diagnosed with throat cancer shortly after I finished treatment, and was subsequently off work himself. I was not ready to return to a job which is challenging, fast paced, and emotionally demanding, and I burnt out quickly, subsequently affecting my mental health.

When I did speak to my doctor following treatment, he – surprisingly – had me on an eight-week return to work plan as I was a 'partner' (thus self-employed), so it was felt there would be more pressure for me to return to work my usual hours. In my vulnerable state, I agreed, and went along with the plan. As we know, healing and recovery are not linear and things didn't work out that way, leaving me feeling like even more of a failure, spiralling down into a hole.

There were days of light, where I absolutely felt I had everything under control. I'd journal that on some days I just 'nailed it'. On the converse, there were times I remember burning out and struggling at work as my hours gradually increased from half days to full, to an increase in the number of days. Every increase in time spent at work or an increase in intensity of work adds a new dimension that precipitates a drop in energy levels and an increase in fatigue, hindering recovery at times. As I've said before, recovery is not linear and nor is your return to work, and understanding this yourself, as well as communicating it to your team, can help set realistic expectations for yourself and your employer.

Taking the plunge

I remember sitting across the meeting table with my GP partners, three months after treatment ended, to discuss my thoughts about returning to work. As soon as I opened my mouth, I sobbed, and felt quite unprofessional. However, I felt it was necessary as I recited a list of all the reasons I was worried about returning to work. I was honest, and I needed them to know, because on the outside I looked fine. Even as doctors, unless you have trodden a similar path, it is difficult to fully comprehend the fear and anxiety. They were extremely supportive, and we agreed a flexible return to work at my pace, and I was filled with very mixed emotions about returning. Anxious – will I remember anything? Will I cry? What if I need the toilet in the middle of a consultation? Excited – with possible glimpses of the return of the old me, the doctor, not a patient.

The big day arrived, and I remember returning to work and initially completing paperwork, looking at blood reports and documents that needed review. I had horrendous sciatica so could only stand, which was relentlessly tiring in itself. I needed the toilet constantly. I remember feeling overwhelmed that everyone wanted to say hello and see how I was doing. It was heart-warming but it was also exhausting. I had spent so much time alone recently, I just wanted to hide.

When I read the first oncology letter for a patient with stage 4 bowel cancer who initially had stage 3, seeing they needed a redo of their anterior resection (the same operation I had) for local recurrence brought tears to my eyes. As I read through the letter, every word jumped out of the page at me and I digested the contents in slow motion. I cried for an hour later that evening, with my husband talking me through my own scans and histology (not helpful, I know), as I frantically sat there trying to work out my risk of recurrence, when we knew there was no obvious reason or clear cause.

My husband gently reassured me that local recurrence is rare. But it triggered my fear, a fear that I tried to suppress deep within my brain, a fear that this could be me again.

I still had my own cancer admin to attend to one day a week and needed to prioritize this. Be it therapy, acupuncture, follow-up appointments, physio, I was adamant that these things came first and had learnt that self-care was of paramount importance. My workplace thankfully understood this, but as I re-entered the world of work, these appointments seemed something of a chore at times, too.

A couple of weeks went by, and I decided that I might be ready to start seeing patients again, after all people-facing work was my passion.

May 2019: spontaneous decisions

Spontaneous decisions occur frequently these days, in this life after cancer. This morning at 6.30 a.m., I texted my practice manager as my sciatica felt slightly easier, and I suggested I come to work and see a few patients … just six, with longer appointment slots, and then do my usual admin tasks.

I think all were surprised but I was determined to see it through. And actually there was no build up to a potential start date of seeing patients in the flesh … just 90 minutes between the text and me being physically at work. I won't lie, my heart was racing and I was anxious. When I announced to my husband I was going to see patients, he said to me supportively, don't worry, just think of all the people that have helped or are helping you, and now you get to go back to helping others today, and if it's not today, it will be another day. This spurred me on no end.

I love my practice – as much as they endure my enthusiasm, they had screened patients to ensure nothing too complex walked through my door and allowed breaks for me to walk round to ease the sciatica, go to the toilet and so on. My first patient had back pain! You couldn't write this stuff sometimes, as we both stood through the consultation. And I loved seeing all the paediatric cases – it came back so easily, maybe because I have children of my own.

Apart from the discomfort (I just couldn't get comfortable), I think it went as well as it could have done, and I wasn't left overwhelmed, as I was expecting. Early days. And I felt alive and pumped with adrenaline! Although I've since crashed with tiredness at home, and since returning, I have questioned myself about my management of the patients I saw today and worrying. However, I think this is natural after a period of time away, when your clinical confidence wanes.

No doubt going into work has increased pain to 8/10 as a result of the drive and trying to sit at a desk … but the high today is most definitely 10/10 in terms of a sense of achievement.

And for today, I'll definitely take that.

It was such a milestone seeing patients again, but with that came the patient encounters setting off countless triggers, which would catch me off guard. After all, the beauty of general practice is that it really is like a box of chocolates – you never quite know what person and problem will walk through the door next, and this unpredictability left me on tenterhooks.

I clearly recall seeing my first patient on that first day of face-to-face appointments. The irony continued, as the first patient presented with rectal bleeding (bleeding from their bottom). The same day, a patient who had had treatment for kidney cancer attended telling me his employer was being inflexible with his work conditions, later terminating his contract and telling him, 'Plenty of people have similar problems and you just have to get on with it' (Barbara Wilson, from Working With Cancer, points out that this is direct discrimination under the Equality Act and is in fact illegal in the UK). If only it were that simple. I felt a deep connection with and empathy for him. We talked about survivorship, ways to move forward with life after cancer, counselling and possibly medication for his mood if things didn't improve.

The next patient remarked, 'Are you that doctor who had cancer?', followed by endless pity and sympathy down the phone, as I tried to hold back the tears, unsuccessfully. It was tiring and fulfilling all at the same time. I wasn't sure how I'd feel one moment to the next, and we had to take each day as it came, and make adjustments.

> Week two finished. Three mornings a week. After a couple of days, I had to resort to working from home as it's more comfortable when you can barely sit. I actually find it easier to focus with less distraction too. Week one was tough, tiring and emotional, but week two seems better. Work has also provided me with a great distraction from the fact I've been told not to exercise currently (bar walking and swimming). All my energy is being ploughed into work and home life. But that's fine. I think these goal posts will have to be adjustable!

The struggle some days was real. The triggers were everywhere, and what I hadn't accounted for was the toll they would take over time. There was my first home visit to one of my elderly patients dying of colorectal cancer, breaking the news to the family that the end was in sight and we would do our utter best to ensure her mother's comfort.

I held her hand and didn't want to let go. Suppressing my own emotions in these situations was energy depleting.

Then there were other heartbreaking stories of those who had lost loved ones to cancer. The woman who had lost her child and husband to cancer, and the patient who had lost their son aged 40 to bowel cancer, then her brother in law and then her husband to stomach cancer all in the same year. Cancer has a lot to answer for. My heart weighed heavy with the emotional burden at times.

I frequently took naps on the patient couch between surgeries (my surgery times were initially a little shorter), as I was so exhausted. And I would crash after a few hours at work, unable to give my family the time they also needed. The guilt and negative self-talk were becoming louder in my head. 'Why can't I just get on with this job?'

I remember digging my nails into the table at my first multidisciplinary palliative care cancer meeting, listening to patients young and old being reeled off. I did everything I could to stay seated but all I wanted to do was run. It was too close to home, and I'd had a glimpse of what really was going on behind closed doors. I was also still petrified that this could be me again.

Patients who declined screening tests for colorectal or breast cancer screening would throw me into a frenzy. Clearly, it is a patient's choice if they are given all the right information to make an informed decision as to whether they want to proceed with a test. Nonetheless, I found it difficult in the early days to comprehend the notion that someone would make a choice not to get checked. Perhaps another sign that I returned to work too soon and just wasn't ready.

I had a cancer survivor who would come in regularly and just cry at me. I have no problem with a therapeutic cry, but I had to use all my might to fight back empathetic tears as, really, I could have been looking in a mirror.

There were certainly days where I asked myself, 'Can I still do this job?'

I found with time I began to desensitize and realized I needed more therapy than just counselling to try to dampen my response to the job at hand. The triggering nature of my job highlighted that indeed I was suffering with PTSD. It was at this point, when I spoke to my counsellor, that we thought it might be in my best interests if

I wanted to carry on working in this trigger-filled setting to receive some formal therapy. This later ended up being trauma-based CBT, which I described earlier in the book. I needed to be able to compartmentalize my work and stop it from causing a massive stress response within my body each time. To allow me to work, and not to develop compassion burnout.

Trauma-based CBT made a huge difference to my ability to work, as did time.

'Time is a great healer'

I would roll my eyes secretly when people made this comment time and time again. Yet here I am, about to say the very same thing. That time does indeed heal, and has continued to help me heal mentally and physically, so my ability to carry out my job without further injury and insult to my wellbeing has improved over the weeks and months.

This doesn't mean that I'm not affected by seeing patients with triggering presentations, but I do not feel the overwhelm as acutely or severely as I previously would have done and I've been able to compartmentalize my job away from my personal experience a little more. I'm well aware, as are my colleagues, that this becomes more onerous around scan times and follow-ups, as I worry about my own health once more. Again, I have found it helpful for myself to inform my colleagues when this time is approaching as my mood and behaviour dip unintentionally. I know then at least I have support during those nerve-wracking times.

So how do you go about returning to work?

After a cancer diagnosis, you are classed as disabled (Equality Act 2010), and many in fact will have an invisible disability. Legally, there should be no unfair discrimination, yet 20 per cent of patients according to one survey experienced this. As I say, transparency about your condition is paramount in the hope that appropriate workplace adjustments can then be made. I appreciate, though, that this is difficult for many, and these conversations can feel personal and sometimes awkward. Remember that by law, all this information is confidential. I worried that I would be judged, as I looked 'well', but it was even more reason for me to spell out the issues.

There are several factors to consider when returning to work, and people often ask me how I went back fairly soon after treatment ended.

Firstly: everyone is different. Your circumstances. Your illness. Your physiology. Your treatment. Your job. Your expectations.

Do whatever is right for you. Trust your gut instinct.

And if your return to work doesn't go to plan, revisit the plan, and know that it is absolutely fine to have more time off.

Check your contract to ascertain what your sick leave policy is, how much is paid and unpaid, and how long for. Talk to any union or employment group you are part of to seek advice if needed or any of the organizations listed at the end of this chapter.

Here's an entry from my journal from when I was contemplating my return to work and why I felt it was important to do so:

May 2019

After a lot of thought, I've decided that I need work in my life to give me that extra 'normality' that I'm missing.

To stop me obsessing and trying to control other aspects in my life.
To give me focus.
To rebuild my self-confidence.
To distract.
To give back to a profession that has saved my life.
To see if I can be that doctor again that I once was.
I don't know if I can do my job right now.
Emotionally.
But if I don't try, I won't know.
And there may never be a right time.
Physically I'm left with mild anaemia from the chemo, a peripheral neuropathy (nerve pains in my feet more than my hands), the sciatica (I cannot sit for any length of time without a searing pain down my left leg), fatigue, concentration difficulties. Not to forget bowel trouble – the frequency and urgency of needing the toilet at times – not the most conducive to good patient care if I'm in the middle of a consultation. Mentally – well that's a can of worms that I'll continue to work through with the counsellor tomorrow. And this is my biggest battle right now. Let's start this ball rolling.

Below is a (non-exhaustive) list of things to think about on returning to work, the workplace you left before cancer:

- Have an open and honest conversation with your employer/HR representative three to four weeks prior to your return if you have been off work for a significant length of time. It may be a difficult and upsetting conversation but most employers do want to help. Your employer is likely to be nervous, too, with a fear of not saying the right thing! Meet with them, take someone with you if need be. Write down any questions you wish to discuss beforehand and perhaps speak to your doctor to discuss a potential return to work. Know your rights, the legislation and research any support out there. Lay all your cards out on the table so that, from the offset, things have been clear to minimize miscommunication. There may be some negotiation but as long as the plan seems reasonable, and your employer has time to adapt and prepare, it may actually lessen the load on yourself as anxiety about return to work can weigh heavily. You may even feel positive about your return. This doesn't work for everyone, and I once had an A&E sister contact me to tell me she had stage 4 cancer, was working with this and didn't want her employers to know as she didn't want to be treated differently. Managing shifts together with treatment was a mine-field but it worked for her, and that's ok, too.

- Talk about specific symptoms that may cause worry or problems and may require more breaks such as toileting, stoma emptying, medication breaks, panic attacks, fatigue, and so on, as well as the need for ongoing appointments or treatment.

- Agree a return to work plan. Have the discussion documented and ensure everyone has a copy including yourself. Keep it flexible and agree to meet to review at regular intervals.

- Decide whether you would like your colleagues in the workplace to know and decide what you would like to tell them, how and when. For example, is it better for them to all know before you start working, so any chat, questions can be dealt with before you focus your energy on the job at hand when you start? Will that information be sent by the line manager on a group email? Think about how you would like this information disseminated and what you would like them to say.

- Plan for a slow and steady return to work on amended hours (a shorter working day initially), amended duties (the job specification may have to change if there are tasks you are unable to do post cancer), or a phased return initially (where you start on a couple of days, rather than five days a week if that was your usual work pattern before cancer).

- Ask for feedback (review and validation – I needed to know I was doing ok – which in turn will help your self-confidence at work grow too, which can often be lacking when you first return).
- Ensure you plan rest into your working week. This may mean sacrificing other activities.
- If it gets too much, keep communication open with colleagues, and let them know.
- Ask family and friends for support as this is a big milestone. Keep the dialogue going about how you're feeling and whether you require extra support with tasks at home.
- Keep in touch with your doctor for any support needed mentally or physically or for sick notes for a phased return to work. If your workplace has an Occupational Health department, it is worthwhile booking an appointment with them as they can help facilitate your return.
- In the UK, Macmillan, Maggie's and Working With Cancer have fantastic resources and support concerning return to work (see Useful Resources), especially if you find yourself in a situation where your employers or HR team aren't so flexible. I've been witness to this a number of times in general practice, too, and I do feel for individuals when employers are unsympathetic or lack the understanding to help. Most of us do want to return to work, and have purpose!
- You'll find further links and resources at the end of this book in Useful Resources.
- And finally, do not rush back to work. Your mental and physical health are the priority.

Many people, including those closest to me, thought I went back to work prematurely. Did I? Probably. However, it gave me a sense of self-worth and allowed my confidence to build up slowly. I was no longer just a patient, wife or mother, I was back in the hot seat as a doctor, ready to help others and give back to those who needed care themselves, and importantly having flexibility offered me a safety net when at times it was all too much.

Working through cancer

Some people are able to work through cancer, despite the mental and physical challenges, and some find themselves having to continue work for financial reasons. If you decide you would like to continue working, flexibility will be required around good and bad days and a reduction of hours or amendment of duties may be necessary depending on the type of job – but the self-help list above still applies. It is important to have insight into what is realistic, and to have honest conversations with your team. Do what is right for you.

The Macmillan and WWC websites have lots of advice regarding returning to work, working through cancer. Having financial pressures and concerns on top of illness is another challenge posed by cancer that can have detrimental effects on a person's wellbeing in a multitude of ways.

What if I can't go back to my job?

Indeed, there may be some who are unable to return to the job they did previously because of the effects of cancer and its treatment limiting their ability to fulfil their duties. If you still wish to work at your previous establishment, do speak to your employer first to see if there are any other roles or adaptations that could be made.

Alternatively, your new perspective may result in a change in direction, and you may want to explore alternative career pathways. Certainly one of my close friends quit her job in London and became a nurse after tending to her husband with cancer. Or if you are able, you may choose to retire early through ill health. WWC provides career coaching to those thinking about changing their job.

What if I'm self-employed or financially stretched?

Unfortunately, not everyone has income protection or critical illness cover, or cover through their workplace. In the USA, not everyone has medical cover or insurance. The added burden of financial stress can be immense and it is so important to seek advice and support.

If you are self-employed, there is not only the financial stress if you are unable to work, but also fear for the business that you have built up. On the other hand, if you're able to continue working, you may be able to do so flexibly. Macmillan again has a whole host of support on its website (see Useful Resources).

In summary, work and cancer may conjure up a whole manner of emotions, from the guilt of not firing on all cylinders and being unable to fulfil all your previous duties, to the need for time off for appointments. It can feel frustrating that you cannot work as you used to BC and work may not seem as fulfilling. You may worry what others think or how they will react and frankly there is a lot to think about. It is a whole different aspect of your life, requiring time and support.

The bottom line is to keep communication lines open with your employer (if you have one), or those around you, put your wellbeing (physical and mental) first and, if you are struggling, seek help and adjust the goal posts set out, and remember these are, and should be, movable. Seek support – the Useful Resources section at the back of the book has a wealth of resources signposting access to help when it comes to working with and after cancer.

19

What cancer gave me – life with and after cancer

Cancer can feel like it takes a lot away, but it can also give back in ways you never expected.

A study from 2019 looked at stage 2 and stage 3 breast cancer patients and showed that cancer survivors showed mostly positive changes in themselves and life after cancer.

I started writing the positive changes cancer had brought to my life in a bid to try to gain more clarity in my head about my own feelings and identity post cancer. During this time, I'd learnt a lot about myself but also about others, and knew there have been some positive life changes that cancer has brought with it.

Recently, during a talk I was giving on 'Moving forwards after cancer', I asked a group of young adult cancer survivors to write down the positives cancer had given them, to try to turn the negative narrative on its head, and to help them grow and indeed move forwards after cancer. They all were able to come up with a few things, just showing that if we turn our mindset and fine tune it, we can try to make lemonade out of the basket of lemons that has been hurled at us.

For me, there are also all the positives cancer has brought to my personal and professional life, and I've gained so much in terms of personal growth, wisdom and clarity during life after cancer. I've learnt that it's ok not to be ok, to show vulnerability, to make mistakes and to live life to the full, and take nothing for granted, especially my health.

It really is a double-edged sword.

Here's Emma's perspective (as a stage 4 bowel cancer survivor) on 'what cancer gave me' and the power of positivity:

Emma

At the start of my journey, my best friend would sometimes send me quotes. Quotes about positivity or strength. She knows me well, so she knows I have a good sense of humour (somewhat amplified since cancer as well – if you don't laugh you'll cry…) and one of these quotes she sent me, back in 2020, just stuck. Something clicked inside me when I read it, it was deep, I could relate, it had a strong message but it also made me laugh!

'Being negative only makes a journey more difficult. You may be given a cactus but you don't have to sit on it!'

Joyce Meyer

And this became my mantra, and cacti became my 'thing'. Even now, people send me little things with cacti on, and if I am out shopping and I see something with a cactus on it, I have to have it. When I got my first all clear, despite it being lockdown, we had a little party at home, just the five of us… it was a cactus party with cactus decorations and home-made cactus-themed snacks. Even my children now know 'mum likes cacti' and will point them out. This quote, and seeing cacti, reminds me that we are all dealt crap hands in life; some more crappy than others. But how we deal with it, really, can be the making or breaking of a situation. Do I believe being positive will cure my cancer, or anybody else's? No. I believe in science and medicine, but I do believe that being positive can help the way you feel, and that when I feel bad emotionally, and I go into a bad place, I almost make myself physically ill. So, there is a link, I think, between the physical and mental states of a person; I can't control the physical so much (although I have tried with diet, exercise and lifestyle changes since cancer) but I can control the mental. And I certainly ain't sitting on my cactus, I can tell you that!

Conversely, I also know this is not always easy, and I've seen some patients never feel any of the positives from their circumstances, too.

The negatives can stay at the forefront at times, especially when we are suffering with physical limitations, or the mental pain and anguish still command all our attention. As we navigate this roller-coaster, it feels more gratifying to focus on any positives, and to let these negative moments be exactly that. Just a moment.

Post-traumatic growth

I decided to write my own 'what cancer gave me list', and realized inadvertently that I was describing the gifts of post-traumatic growth. There is no doubt that growth can be painful, but to see the brightest lights, we sometimes have to venture through the darkest moments and, as a result of trauma, I've received the gifts below by conquering adversity. Following therapy, the time that has passed since diagnosis, the moments of reflection and tears and having had the courage to witness, process and accept my terror, cancer most definitely has now witnessed me grow as a person.

Post-traumatic growth describes the transformation post trauma or stress and the five domains of post-traumatic growth include:

- New possibilities and opportunities
- Closer relationships
- Increased personal strength
- Greater appreciation for life
- Spiritual development

They can include things such as finding God, writing a book (I'll put my hand up to this one), setting up a charity, quitting your job for a job you actually want to do, and so on. For each of these domains, I have written down examples from my own experience – a really useful exercise for anyone facing trauma, or a life-changing event, to try to move positively forwards after an event.

New possibilities and opportunities

- An education – I have learnt so much about not only myself, but also about this disease and everything that goes with it.
- More spontaneity, meaning that we are making so many memories together and experiencing what some may experience in a decade, all rammed into a year – although I fear I exhaust my friends and family with this some days.
- Accepting my new normal, and learning to live with this, yet still knowing the world is my oyster.
- Experiencing incredible highs and taking on new experiences that may have never come my way; pursing new challenges that I never thought I could ever achieve in my wildest dreams. These include writing this book, running the London Marathon (after being told 18 months previously that I may never run more than 5 km again due to sciatica), working for a wide range of charities in various capacities (fundraising, raising awareness, as a media and medical opinion volunteer, becoming a trustee to Teens Unite and patron to the Fountain Centre, the very charity that helped my family through the shit and beyond).

- Working in the media, as a TV doctor, involvement in a variety of campaigns supporting cancer awareness, health education or health promotion, as well as breaking down taboos and stigma-laden topics, including women's health.

Closer relationships

- Gaining new friends who do just 'get it', and I always feel enveloped in the hugest comfort blanket when I finally meet these people in real life (my Insta gang and my cancer friends).
- Finding out who you can rely on, those unshakeable individuals who will be true to you, be your biggest cheerleaders and enjoy watching you grow and morph into that person after cancer. I can safely say I have relationships that have blossomed, strengthened and become unbreakable since cancer.
- I am less tolerant of people shirking away, not behaving appropriately or hurting my feelings, and I'm not afraid to call people out on that, without (hopefully) being rude!
- I truly understand what impact a doctor can make to a patient's day or life – that a negative experience can last a lifetime, and a positive experience gives you the feeling that 'you've got this', and someone else has your back, 100 per cent.
- A deeper empathy and understanding for those who are having a difficult time – whatever that may be. My compassion has also increased as I find myself switching between patient and doctor.

Increased personal strength

- Tenacity and resilience – when I get knocked down, I get up again, and again, and again, ploughing on even when I don't feel like it. I've developed and felt a strength (physically and mentally) within myself that I never thought I had, overcoming obstacle after obstacle, getting back on that horse every time I fell off and trying to make the best of whatever life has thrown at me.
- On reflection, I've seen how brave I can be, and it's given me courage to pursue things I would have never considered previously.
- I'm finding the courage to start saying no, so I focus on the things I have wanted to say yes to, thereby concentrating my efforts on things that fire a passion.

- I've opted for more self-care and self-preservation as I've accepted it was imperative not only for recovery, but actually for day-to-day life.
- I'm astonished and proud of what my body can do, how it can heal and what it has seen me through.

Greater appreciation for life

- My appreciation for the smaller things in life is so much greater, and these things give me far more fulfilment and pleasure than I've ever felt previously.
- A greater appreciation of the beautiful world we live in and the people around me, while feeling at the same time more present. The blue skies. The sunsets. Nature.
- Gratitude – for all things big and small. For example, if I only needed the toilet once that day and I was pain free, this was a huge win sometimes and something I would be utterly grateful for.
- Not sweating the small stuff.
- Having more of a 'Does it really matter?' attitude about issues that may have stressed me out in the past.
- Making memories has always outweighed material possessions but even more so now, a greater sense of what really is important in life.
- And last but not least, valuing every day. The good days, the bad days, every day is a gift.

Spiritual development

I was brought up Hindu; unfortunately for me, any belief that I may have had in God has now vanished and, speaking to Danni, she tells me this isn't uncommon. However, some people find comfort in their faith, and some tell me they find deeper meaning in life way beyond the confines of space, time and the universe.

There is also another gift that cancer brings to the table.

The Cancer Card

The Cancer Card will be presented to you along with your new found cancer status – take it. Use it wisely. Some of you may be thinking 'what on earth is a 'Cancer Card? Are there loyalty points or free gifts? Is it so you can obtain treatment?'

In fact, none of the above. The Cancer Card is almost like a 'get out of jail free' card, as coined by those affected with cancer. The user keeps the card in their wallet at ALL times and brings it out on an as-needed basis. What is special about this card is that it trumps everything. What is interesting is that, when this imaginary card arrives, no one knows quite what to do with it. Until, one day, it comes into its own.

November 2019

It was a dreary day. I had dragged my chemo-laden body to a 'Look Good, Feel Better' course that frankly I had no energy for. Yet I had the most inspiring and engaging time attending. I came out of the course with a tiny bounce in my step, with a face full of make-up and goodies, to see the hospital ticket warden by my car. My chemo head swimming, I panicked. Did I pay for a car parking ticket? Did I? I just couldn't remember. And in one quick swoop, the Cancer Card was presented, brand new and shiny, ready to cash in. To my amazement, as I waffled on about my cancer, chemo and chemo brain (to the point I think I drove the traffic warden to boredom or frightened him away), there it was. No ticket. No fine. And just like that, the Cancer Card was played. Cha-ching, cashed in. This wouldn't be the last time.

Humour is required at times when faced with adversity. The Cancer Card certainly gave us an element of this, although there is nothing funny about being diagnosed with cancer. However, where I could, I did try to get through times with as much humility and humour as possible, and my friends teased me as the card was still pulled out on an as and when required basis.

The Cancer Card can highlight to others exactly what a struggle cancer and its treatment can be, a reality that is an education in itself.

Confession time: what have I used the Cancer Card for?

- If I'm too tired, it gives me a free pass to pull out, or go back to bed. Get out of chores, get out of seeing people.
- An excuse to shop. (On one occasion I bought three pairs of trainers, to my husband's utter bewilderment, because I WILL get back to running and these trainers WILL help me, even if I wear a pair on my hands.)
- For forgetting deadlines, birthdays, school admin.
- For getting upgraded on a plane as I couldn't sit up straight for hours due to sciatica so I was offered a lie-flat seat in first class.
- Jumping the toilet queue.

The card does come with two warnings: it may not always be successful, and do not overuse! Most cancer Muggles are unaware that you are using it, but if you repeatedly try to use it, you may find they wise up to it and reject your card!

As well as the above, cancer offers the following ...

Cancerversary

A cancerversary is a milestone defined by YOU. Be it the day you were diagnosed, the day you or your loved one had surgery and had the tumour removed, the day treatment ended, or anything else significant to you for that matter.

Everyone is so different when it comes to their cancerversary. Some want to lay low, and forget the day ever existed. For me, it's not a day to celebrate or commiserate but to just be. I try to remember what I said the day I was diagnosed. I vowed to turn a negative into a positive and to raise awareness from that day forth, ensuring I used my position as a medic and patient to form a platform, and reflect back on what I have achieved.

Reaching milestones

I use milestones like this to reflect on how far I've come, but everyone's milestones will be different. I definitely see birthdays as milestones more than I did before cancer. These milestones can be evocative, and reproduce feelings of grief for what life was before, but also for everything you have been through, celebrating that you have the privilege of having one more year alive, the most precious commodity ever.

As time has gone on, I see clear scans as milestones and those living with cancer find that stable scans are also such pivotal moments after a diagnosis of cancer. And as time has rolled on, I've felt compelled to celebrate these moments too. After all, we should celebrate life. More life, a ticket to health for the next however many months till the next scan, and hopefully so much more. You cannot, honestly, ever put a price on that.

How do you live positively after a life-changing illness/event or cancer?

One of the questions I am most asked, and this is not an easy one to answer as it's so personal.

What I will say is that you can be positive, and think positively, without always feeling happy or optimistic. You're totally entitled to down days too, which I also experience, where the noise of cancer can drown out everything else.

Top 10 tips for living positively

1 **Compartmentalize:** Don't let your imagination run away with you; try to stay in the here and now. Open the 'cancer box' when needed. Sometimes it does open without permission!

2 **Find your tribe:** Your support network. Appreciate your tribe and hold on tight to them.

3 **Live for the moment:** Practise gratitude, and focus on the here and now.

4 **Turn negatives into positives:** This is not for everyone but many choose to turn their hand to fundraising, working with charities, sharing experiences and supporting others, raising awareness.

5 **Relish new opportunities:** Those that you may not have taken up or been offered before.

6 **Plan fun things or make plans:** Making plans after cancer is very daunting initially especially as you swing from scan to scan in an abyss. But for me, it also serves as a distraction. I'm also far more spontaneous, especially when the cancer box opens.

7 **Celebrate every win:** Big or small. From getting back to the gym to running a marathon. From getting the chemo down you when you really don't want to, to the clear scans. Every birthday, every milestone. Make it count. As my nearest know, I don't need much of an excuse to celebrate these days!

8 **Focus:** On the things you can control.

9 **Therapy:** This was pivotal to my recovery and outlook.

10 **Exercise:** The power of exercise is multifactorial.

Gratitude

As clichéd as it may sound, this is one of the things cancer has given me in abundance. It is very much a coping mechanism and facilitates dealing with the negative impact of cancer. Clearly it is difficult to be grateful during treatment, there can be some very heavy and dismal days.

Genuinely, though, I'm so grateful to be alive, to see another day, another sunset or sunrise, to be able to hold my family, to get back to work, for all the treatment and health professionals involved in my care. Because when you stare down a rifle barrel hearing the words 'you have cancer', and face your own mortality prematurely, there is nothing quite like it to give you a kick up the backside, to say 'wake up, smell the coffee, you're alive'. And yes, life can be incredibly tough, but we have to try to embrace each day as best we can, and be thankful for something, even on the worst days. Because if you think about it hard enough, there's always something you can be thankful for.

We also know that gratitude can help facilitate personal growth, with healing and positivity. Studies have also shown that feeling thankful can improve your mood, help with anxiety and depression, improve sleep and your immune system, and reduce chronic pain, so plenty to be thankful about there!

Speaking to so many patients through work or through the cancer community, living positively after cancer is not aways easy, so please don't feel guilty or feel negatively about yourself. It may be that you need to speak to a health professional if suggestions from the list above are not helping. If you feel that each day is persistently negative or a 'red' day, and it is affecting your mood, it may be that professional help is required.

Social media

I always wanted to take my cancer diagnosis and run with it wherever it took me. As a doctor, I needed to help others who found themselves in the same boat and I wanted to drive early diagnosis and prevention.

I set up an Instagram account with my best friend who had been cajoling me to do this for some time. So, while she sat with me waiting to see my cancer specialist nurse, Angie, she set up the account. 'It will help you and it will help others,' she said encouragingly, knowing me at that point far better than I knew my shadow of a self. I was unsure – I was not a big social media user, had no idea what I was doing and wasn't sure if people were even really that interested or whether it would help me. And lo and behold, it became my catharsis, a source of education, a way to raise awareness and a community that supported me as well as others.

My Instagram account has grown organically. I didn't see myself as a writer, but cancer certainly brought out the writer in me, where words flowed thick and fast as a waterfall, and my emotions poured out. This journalling, this writing, this reflecting, it became so therapeutic, a bandage for my wounded soul, Social media has been a love/hate relationship at times if I'm honest, and there are times where it helped my progress and other times where it has dented my self-confidence. I don't understand the algorithms and some days I wonder what one earth I'm doing on there. However, as time goes on, it's provided a platform, opening up opportunities, and creating a community for me and for others as we talk about all sorts, from women's health, to cancer awareness, to mental health – and I'd like to think I've been honest through the process. And I know that this is all worth doing, if I can help even one person out there.

The cancer community – 'Do I want to be part of this gang?'

I couldn't write this chapter without talking about the safety blanket that cancer gifted me, the one that is always there. Even if it's just hanging up in the background, at times of need it is a mighty powerful tool and one that makes you feel so held. The people I am referring to are those who have been afflicted by cancer, and whom I've met online through social media platforms like Instagram. These individuals have taught me so much, spurred me on during times of self-doubt, encouraged me, praised me, supported me, lifted me up during dark times and comforted me, almost as if I've known them for years.

Connecting with people in this way is not for everyone, but it helped me make sense of what was happening, and I felt truly seen and less alone.

Even though I had my own team behind me it felt exhausting, and even futile some days, trying to explain why you felt a certain way or struggled the way you did, and at times my feelings could be invalidated unintentionally.

Some of my pre-cancer friends really couldn't understand why I wanted to be involved in this community once treatment ended and even two or three years down the line. As I say, cancer never totally leaves, and even more so with my job. Even if it is put in its box, somewhere, at some point, it emerges, uninvited. I also genuinely want to use my experience to help others, to help them try to make sense of what can be a bewildering and frightening time.

I can't explain the unbreakable, strong wrought iron bonds that form between fellow cancer patients, they just do. An unspoken, mutual understanding. Many of these people I have never met in real life, but it is totally overwhelming when that moment arrives, as you follow their stories, their achievements, their setbacks, and become so emotionally invested as you travel on each other's rollercoasters, together. I wouldn't have all the wonderful contributors to this book, if it wasn't for social media.

And this, for some people, may be the exact reason for not wanting to be involved in such a community. For one thing, the loss in the community – well, it hits hard. It hurts. It's painful and my heart breaks when another family is ripped apart. And some months the losses come thick and fast and there are times self-preservation is required, and you have to look away. For other people, forming these sorts of relationships may prevent them from moving on with their life after cancer too, something I know those around me worry about.

Again, there is no right or wrong in terms of whether you choose to become part of a community or not, but I'm sharing this as an option for support that you may indeed find useful.

Raising awareness

For me, raising awareness was an extension of my day job. I spend a lot of my time on health promotion and I can see the gaps with clear lenses, post cancer: where work needs to happen, and where we need to raise awareness.

I also accept that cancer is part of my tapestry and although day to day, any negative feelings from cancer are somewhat dampened, I do feel that any daily reminders of cancer are curbed by the positivity I try to generate through my work.

For others, the desire is to leave cancer life behind as much as they can. To carry on with the new normal and to live life as best as one can in between scans and surveillance. I'm not saying this is easy, however, I can totally see the advantage of this some days when cancer can consume my every waking hour, for example writing this book – or during scan time. Wouldn't it be nice to not talk about cancer some days? On the whole, as I've explained to friends who have questioned my apparent need to keep talking about cancer, for me it just never leaves. This is not only seen in the daily side effects of surgery and treatment, but also as a result of my work. Day after day, I see patient after patient, trying to assess – does this patient have cancer? A sea of constant red flags waving in my mind.

One of the hardest things about raising awareness and being part of the community is being a doctor myself. So many people (especially those younger) have been diagnosed late with colorectal cancer, feeling fobbed off by their doctor, unseen and unheard, and initially, I took any statements made to heart, trying to protect a profession I work in, wanting to explain the complex factors for this. To explain that, at med school, we were taught that CRC was, classically, a disease of overweight, white males, aged 60 or over.

However, as I listened to more and more stories, it became clear there was a lot of work that needed to be done in terms of increasing awareness of bowel cancer in the young, something many were unaware of, let alone with an increasing incidence - so there was a need for re-education. And as doctors, we are always learning and expected to keep up to date. And it was clear that there was a common complaint – that doctors needed to LISTEN. As doctors, the most important duty we have is to listen. Even if I think a patient's medical complaint is unlikely to result in any serious pathology, that patient should be able to express their ideas, concerns and expectations, and feel listened to.

As a result, I found myself trying to raise awareness of bowel cancer in the young within bodies of health professionals, be it giving lectures to medical trainees or junior doctors, or by sharing my story on social media and on doctors' platforms, all of which are received well, often with thanks for highlighting this, or prompting discussions of cases so we can all learn from one another.

Opportunity knocks

For a while after treatment, where there was no way I could contemplate doing any more than getting through the day, and pushing the boundaries into pastures new would fuel anxiety levels as I wondered if I would physically, emotionally and mentally manage opportunities presented, and imposter syndrome would creep in. My own self-confidence at the time was rock bottom, and my vulnerability and fragility levels were sky-high. I was also torn between my burning desire to engage in philanthropic work versus trying to be a mother, wife and a doctor once more. As time elapsed after treatment ended, I did in fact manage to fulfil my desire and work on a variety of campaigns and for charities, which in itself was exhilarating and exhausting in equal measures. My GP mentor, who was allocated to me on my return from sick leave, would quite often tell me how my face lit up the room as soon as I started talking about cancer awareness or working with charities, and that my passion was palpable.

Being part of these campaigns did wonders for my self-confidence and helped me overcome some of the anxiety I faced post cancer. With one photoshoot for The C-List, I had photos bearing my port scar for the first time for all to see. I never really exposed it, I hadn't been able to touch it for months without cringing and had completed some work with my therapist to manage this.

Following this, and discussing my interest in awareness work with an online friend called H, who worked for a UK show called *Lorraine*, I was asked to appear on *Lorraine* and on the national news to join the 'No Butts' campaign, raising awareness for bowel cancer, set up by the legend, the late Dame Deborah James and the *Lorraine* team. It was and still is a cheeky but serious campaign, one that I was honoured to be part of, and continue to be so. The aim of this campaign was to 'break the poo taboo, to wipe away the stigma, flush away the stigma and get the nation talking about poo' – and this is what my husband and I talked at length about – the countless lives this campaign could save. Times were definitely changing.

This led to further work as a media doctor, working in various forums trying to raise awareness of a variety of topics as well as bowel cancer.

All this work and all these opportunities have been incredibly rewarding. In all honesty, I've just wanted to share my unique position as a doctor and as a patient giving back in whatever capacity I can, hoping that my work and intentions indeed make a difference.

20

Cancer within communities

Being from an ethnic minority and cancer – the challenges

The perception of cancer in ethnic minority groups can be filled with shame, taboo, stigma and even, at times, ignorance. Family members with a cancer diagnosis can be silenced or worse still ousted, and they can be made to feel the cancer was their fault or even God's will. Cancer can be deemed 'contagious' or a curse, for example, in Black ethnic minority groups and in South Asian groups, cancer is a condition which isn't often spoken about, is kept as a 'secret' among the immediate family members, and is associated with fear and embarrassment.

Being Asian, I was fortunate that I didn't feel the taboo and stigma, partly because I'm a doctor, and partly because of the way I have been brought up. However, I've heard many stories of others within the community who choose to openly talk about their diagnosis or raise awareness being shunned or spoken badly of. There are also not many people of colour representing those with cancer in the public eye. Diversity and representation are so important, in order for all individuals to be represented and 'seen', and to make people think, this indeed could happen to them. This is one of the many reasons I have chosen to speak up about bowel cancer, fly this flag, and bring my perspective to the table – to push boundaries and break the stereotype, showing others that there is nothing to be ashamed about and we can support one another.

There are also well-documented health inequalities when it comes to cancer diagnosis and care in ethnic minority groups. This is something we need to work hard at to improve. By raising awareness, we strive for change and open the dialogue that we need to do better for all communities and groups of people, any of whom can be afflicted by cancer.

Studies and data so far highlight that ethnic minority groups:

- have lower symptom awareness – so need targeted cancer awareness campaigns
- are more likely to present late with cancer and not seek help initially
- are less likely to attend screening programmes for colorectal, cervical and breast cancer
- have increased difficulties accessing services and an increase in practical and emotional barriers. Practical barriers include juggling other responsibilities such as being a carer, or work, and 'not having time', and there are also language barriers to consider. Emotional barriers include lack of confidence to see a doctor and fear. When interviewing Danni our psychotherapist, she tells me of her experiences with the therapy she provides – that only a handful of those from ethnic communities come forward for counselling and when they do, it is often in a 'discreet' or hidden manner. 'I can't tell my family I'm here having counselling, they told me to keep it all within the community or family.' The notion is that cancer should be kept secret
- face a paucity of data relating to prevalence and cancer experiences due to a lack of studies on, and enrolment in studies of, individuals from ethnic minorities. This may also be due to mistrust of health professionals and researchers
- tend to have unknown family history (if cancer wasn't spoken about)
- have a lack of awareness regarding risk factors for CRC
- are poorly understood by healthcare providers in terms of cultural differences and the needs of black and minority ethnic groups due to the shame and stigma a cancer diagnosis can bring in these groups
- have more negative experiences in terms of patient satisfaction compared with white groups
- are more likely to suffer depression following cancer, many withholding their feelings from their families and not disclosing their illness even to their children.

Teasing things apart further, the following reasons for such barriers may include:

- Fear of cancer or the screening process
- The belief that cancer doesn't happen to people in their community
- Embarrassment/shame – fear of being an outcast
- Taboo – not appropriate to talk about it culturally
- Cultural myths and perceptions – for example, witches and witchcraft can be used to transmit cancers, Western medicine or hospital treatment may worsen cancers, talking about cancer may enhance its power
- Language barriers
- Lack of awareness and health education
- Religious beliefs
- Cultural beliefs.

So, what can we do to promote change?

- Talk about this openly – address the issues and misinformation.
- Patient education – providing information in a variety languages (the NHS indeed do this). Go out into communities and educate.
- Spread the word and share information about screening programmes and tests in a positive light.
- Identify the specific ethnic groups for which risk factor and screening awareness are low.
- Talk within communities, speaking to children openly about bodily functions, educating them at school.
- Target areas with low uptake – programmes rolled out by the NHS with professional health facilitators who can phone patients or speak to groups – speak to them in their language and address any concerns.
- Educate health professionals – understanding cultural beliefs and perceptions can help challenge these. Research ways of debunking myths and misconceptions.
- Ask leaders in the community, imams, or leaders at the temple, to hold forums to discuss health awareness and screening (separate talks for men and women).
- Encourage people from ethnic minorities to take part in research so we can help address health inequalities and lack of data in these sub-groups.

There are support groups again on Facebook and a UK-based charity called Black Women Rising which has a fantastic website full of resources, a magazine and podcast to help give ethnic minorities a space when it comes to cancer (see Useful Resources).

Bowel cancer and the LGBTQ+ community

Here, LGBTQ+ includes all those who identify as lesbian, bisexual, gay, transgender, queer or intersex. As well as within ethnic minority groups, there are huge health inequalities when it comes to cancer experience in the LGBTQ+ community. Again, there are a number of reasons for this:

- Lack of data and cancer registries providing sexual orientation information, as well as a lack of studies.
- There are a number of barriers, including fear of discrimination about their sexual orientation, leading individuals to be worried that their sexual orientation may impact the care offered. However, evidence suggests disclosure of sexual identity and acceptance of the disclosure by health professionals is associated with improved patient satisfaction and patient outcomes.
- Lower rates of health insurance in the USA within the LGBTQ+ community due to higher rates of homelessness, mental health issues, and higher rates of unemployment. Some insurance policies do not cover unmarried partners, leading to difficulties in accessing care and therefore potentially delaying diagnosis (according to the American Cancer Society). Negative experiences with healthcare providers or the fear of a negative experience can discourage individuals from coming forward when they have symptoms, or to complete screening tests.
- CRC survivorship is often understudied and not spoken about as much and, until 2017, there were no studies looking at survivorship among LGBTQ+ individuals. This study suggested that there was a significant economic impact on LGBTQ+ individuals that could indeed affect survivorship. Losing a job in the USA also results in a potential loss of health coverage which impacts their future surveillance. Loss of housing is also reported as a social issue due to loss of income, not being able to live alone etc.

Bowel cancer in older people

We know that your risk of colorectal cancer increases with age. Six out of ten cases are in the over 70s, and most of my patients are over 70 when they are diagnosed. At this point we often have to bear in mind their physical and mental health when thinking about treatment options.

I have had conversations with some of my older patients and their families over the years, and below are some of the questions I have been asked.

'Will I get the same treatment as someone 20 years younger?'

Treatment decisions will be based on a multitude of factors – the stage of cancer, your physical health, fitness and exercise tolerance, your medical history and fitness for general anaesthetic if surgery is required (specifically looking at lung, kidney, heart, and liver function), your medications, your social set-up and so much more. Options will then be presented to you by your specialist.

'Do I have to go through the investigations?'

Once in a while, I've been in this situation as a doctor where I have a high clinical suspicion about a patient having a bowel cancer diagnosis. However, the patient or their family member may have stipulated that obtaining a diagnosis would be futile, putting them through an unnecessary burden of tests when actually their quality of life is poor, they are frail, and actually they wouldn't tolerate any treatment. In other words, it wouldn't be in the best interests of the patient to plough forward with investigations for a diagnosis that they are not fit enough to be treated for. In these cases, we aim to keep patients comfortable, not knowing for sure whether there is a cancer, nor the extent of the disease.

'What if I don't want treatment?'

You will have the right to discuss all the options and decide with your specialist team what you feel would be best and what you are willing to go through. No one can force you to have treatment, but they can give you all the information you need to make an informed decision. Questions you may want to ask include:

- What will treatment entail?
- What are the advantages of having treatment? Is there a survival advantage?
- What are the side effects? How will treatment affect me day to day physically and mentally?
- What are the alternatives?
- How will my medical history and medication affect my treatment?
- If I don't have treatment, will you keep monitoring me?

'My mother has dementia. We don't want her to go through the process.'

There are occasions when patients are unable to make decisions for themselves, such as with dementia.

Sometimes there may be an LPA (lasting power of attorney) for health and welfare (which is totally separate from a LPA for property and financial affairs). This will stipulate that you are able to make medical decisions on your relative's behalf.

If there isn't an LPA in place, doctors will make a decision taking into consideration your thoughts and wishes, but also taking into account what would be in the best interests of the patient.

'What if my family don't respect my wishes?'

This situation can arise when family members, for example, would like their loved one to take up all the treatment options in the hope of prolonging life or, conversely, do not want their loved one to have treatment due to concerns about their physical and mental wellbeing. In these situations, it is best for the family members to talk through their worries with the medical team so all can be addressed.

Bowel cancer in pregancy

Earlier, we met Lauren who presented with colorectal cancer in pregnancy. She is not alone. The diagnosis of CRC in pregnancy can be challenging and complicated, as symptoms may mimic those which occur in pregnancy – anaemia, abdominal pain, constipation, some rectal bleeding from piles, nausea, vomiting and even weight loss. Unfortunately, due to this, patients often present at a more advanced stage. It is the seventh most common cancer presenting in pregnancy and the challenges with CRC and pregnancy will no doubt rise, as the incidence of this cancer increases in the young.

What will happen?

Due to the fact it is a rare presentation, we are limited in terms of data and studies and so a multidisciplinary team including an obstetrician is pivotal when co-ordinating care and deciding treatment options.

It is rare for the foetus to come to any harm from the cancer, but some of the investigations cannot be performed without presenting a risk to the mother or foetus and so, difficult treatment decisions will arise.

If the cancer is detected during the first 20 weeks, discussions regarding termination may occur, as delaying treatment for any length of time may lead to the cancer spreading and increase the risk of the mother dying from cancer.

After 20 weeks, the surgery may be deferred until the foetus is viable and once delivered, surgery can be performed.

Radiotherapy and immunotherapy are not used in pregnancy, due to their effect on the foetus.

Chemotherapy is safer to give in the second and third trimesters, compared with the first, but can be associated with an increased incidence of prematurity, and intra uterine growth retardation (where a foetus does not grow as expected).

You also cannot breastfeed if you're having chemotherapy, as it will pass from your milk to your baby.

The mental strain

Juggling the anguish of a cancer diagnosis, coupled with pregnancy and managing your own health, is no doubt taxing. Bringing new life into the world should be filled with happiness and joy, and may now be marred by the cancer itself.

Mummy's Star (see Useful Resources) is a wonderful charity supporting anyone who is pregnant and finds themselves diagnosed with cancer, and their families. An extremely useful website and source of information for people in an incredibly difficult situation.

21

Bowel cancer screening (BCS)

I couldn't possibly write a book about bowel cancer without mentioning the bowel cancer screening programme (BCSP), which we know SAVE LIVES. In fact, colorectal screening programmes can reduce an individual's risk from dying from CRC by a staggering 25 per cent.

What is screening?

Screening is a way of identifying apparently healthy people (those who have no symptoms), who may be at an increased risk of developing a particular condition. The aim is to offer screening to those who would benefit most from it.

This is crucial in terms of diagnosing not only bowel cancer in the early stages, but importantly the precursors of bowel cancer (polyps), which otherwise remain undetected as they frequently do not produce any symptoms.

Why do we need screening for colorectal cancer?

- It is the second biggest cancer killer in the UK and the USA
- It often presents with no symptoms in the early stages
- It is a potentially treatable and curable cancer if caught early

How do we screen?

The bowel cancer screening test initially sent out in the post is called the faecal immunochemical test, or FIT test for short. FIT tests detect microscopic amounts of blood in the stool which are not visible to the naked eye, and if present, can be a sign of a bowel polyp – or of cancer. FIT tests are also available from pharmacies and can be purchased online, although these use different thresholds for detecting blood than the BCSP does. Clear instructions on how to collect the stool sample are included with the kit, and the test is then returned by post.

Most tests in the BCSP are negative (98 out of 100). If your FIT test is negative (in the UK), you will simply be invited back for a repeat test in two years. If a FIT test comes back as positive, an invite to a specialist screening practitioner appointment will be sent to discuss the result further, at which point an appointment for a diagnostic test (usually a colonoscopy) will be scheduled to take place within two weeks.

In the US, the Cologuard test is used (see Chapter 3) and, if this is positive, a colonoscopy will be offered.

Who do we screen?

In the UK, the national colorectal cancer screening programme was introduced in 2006, initially screening those between the ages of 60–74. However, 94 per cent of bowel cancers are diagnosed in the over 50s. In line with these statistics, recent campaigning by the charity Bowel Cancer UK saw the age limit lowered in the UK and now everyone between the ages of 50 and 74 will eventually be offered a bowel cancer screening test every two years.

If you are 75 and over, you can self-refer into the BCSP every two years by phoning the free bowel cancer screening helpline on 0800 707 6060. Further information can be found on the NHS website.

In the USA, the US Preventive Services Task Force recommends that adults aged 45 to 75 be screened for colorectal cancer. The Task Force recommends that adults aged 76 to 85 consult with their doctor about screening. You can talk to your insurance provider to see what screening you are eligible for. Further information can be found on the American Cancer Society website.

What are the downsides of screening?

Very few. FIT tests are highly sensitive, which means that if a polyp or a cancer is present, the test is highly likely to be positive. They are also specific, which means that if a polyp or cancer is not present, then the test is not likely to be positive. It is important to remember that approximately only 1 in 10 patients with a positive FIT test in the BCSP will be diagnosed with an advanced polyp or a CRC after further tests. A very small proportion of patients participating in the BCSP will be given false reassurance by a negative FIT test when a bowel cancer or polyp is in fact present. But given that no test is 100 per cent perfect, it is important to continue to participate in bowel cancer screening through FIT testing every two years, even if previous tests have been negative and even if you have no symptoms.

This makes sense, so why don't people do it?

Unfortunately, despite all the positives of the BCSP, only 60–70 per cent of patients eligible for screening choose to complete their FIT test kit. Screening uptake tends to be reduced in areas of social deprivation, in males compared to females, and among ethnic minority groups.

The reasons for this are complex, but some of those my colleagues and I have heard before include:

- 'I'm too well to have cancer'
- 'I haven't got time'
- 'The test sounds unpleasant'
- 'There's no history of cancer in my family'
- 'What if it's positive?'
- 'I don't understand what this all means'
- 'It's so embarrassing!'
- 'It won't happen to me'
- 'If it's God's will…'
- 'If it's my time, then it's my time.'

I profess to not fully understanding patients who choose not to participate in cancer screening programmes, and found it difficult to explore their reasons in the early days on my return to work. Whatever the rationale behind their decisions, at the time it seemed nonsensical to me, as my diagnosis had given me a very different perspective. I would have done anything to have had an earlier diagnosis, perhaps avoiding the need to go through chemotherapy, and frankly if my cancer had been detected at the stage of a polyp, I may have avoided surgery and a stoma, too! But each individual is free to make an informed choice regarding their health decisions. There is no doubt that with the passing of time I find it easier to not act as judge

Bowel cancer screening (BCS)

in the matter, but rather I try to explain the rationale and encourage those who choose not to participate.

I remember a 60-year-old man presenting to my surgery, with his bowel cancer screening invite papers, demanding to know 'what all the kerfuffle was about' and 'did he need to do it?' as he felt 'fine'. My own father had even said a very similar thing to me, despite all I had been through! I'll leave it to your imagination as to where the conversation went with both parties from there …

Recently, my sister-in-law's stepfather was diagnosed with colorectal cancer through the screening programme, aged 74. Here he describes his experience. Meet Stan.

Stan

My cancer journey started when a letter from the Bowel Screening Service said they had detected blood in the stool on the screening the test and I would need to go in for a colonoscopy. I wasn't worried, I thought the procedure might be unpleasant, but I was reassured that most people picked up during the screening ended up having haemorrhoids or polyps.

During the colonoscopy I was alert and watching on the screen. It was obvious there was a problem, even I could see a small growth that looked like it was bleeding. The doctor took a biopsy, asked me to phone my wife, and within an hour we were chatting in a small room with him. He said the lesion was almost certainly cancer, but it was very small, about 1 cm, and he was optimistic surgery would cure it. I had a CT scan to see if there was any spread, but all was clear and we were very relieved.

Ten days later we met the surgeon, who explained I would need a right hemicolectomy, an operation to remove the whole right side of my large intestine. He would perform the surgery using robotics, the incision would be small and low down in the abdomen, and there would be three or four other small holes about 6 to 8 mm in diameter. This would make recovery much quicker.

The pre op for the surgery was straightforward though the operation took a little longer than the predicted 3–4 hours. Everything went according to plan – we hadn't realized that 'robotic assisted' means that the surgeon does not even have to be in the operating theatre!

I felt pretty rough the first day. I was well looked after, and started drinking fluids. I had a cannula in my arm through which they gave me my medication, and a catheter for urine. I was linked to a monitor checking my heart rate and oxygen saturation. I had a morphine pump that I could press if I needed a boost of painkillers.

I was doing so well that I was discharged on day three. The next few days I took it easy, walked about the house interspersed with rest and naps. By the end of the week I went for a half mile walk, and within two weeks I would say I was 90 per cent. I hardly had any pain, the incision was healing well, one hole in my

295

abdomen had a large scab, the holes were barely visible. Within three weeks I was driving the car, and walking well. I did avoid strenuous exertion and lifting.

At our daughter's wedding, I was completely back to normal, and able to join in the ceilidh dancing!

I am very grateful for the bowel screening programme and would urge anyone who is offered a test to do it without hesitation. Without it I would not have known there was anything wrong for a long time, as I had no symptoms and no rectal bleeding. Such a simple, easy test, and I am hopeful it has saved my life.

The message regarding screening is simple. Please ensure invites to screening aren't ignored or forgotten, please don't defer it for another day, please check on your friends and family, and remind those closest to you who are eligible for screening programmes to participate in theirs. Encourage open conversations about the programme. In my view, this is a perfectly reasonable subject matter for discussion over the table at a dinner party (yes my husband and I have been known to bring it up – you can expect wild times when you come to dinner with us!) and while I fully appreciate that participating in screening is a personal choice, please ensure it is an informed choice and that you have all the information you need before you make your decision.

Any concerns or questions, talk to your doctor or look online at www.nhs.uk. Believe me, I would choose screening over cancer, ANY day of the week, ANY week of the year, because we know that screening really does save lives.

22

Hope

Claire, age 53, stage 4 thriver

I am living with an abundance of hope. When I lie awake at night, I don't worry about the future, I channel hope and ask why my outcome shouldn't be a good one!

It's incredibly tough, and for me the worst part is seeing my loved ones upset. I'm devastated I'm putting them in this position so I have to stay optimistic because they take their lead from me – that's a lot of effort for me at times but the only way to be. Worrying and ruminating about 'what ifs' is truly pointless. And that doesn't mean I'm not realistic – if I make it to octogenarian status then that will be a miracle but with research and treatment advances why shouldn't I hope for that?

My aim is to enjoy every day, to be grateful for every day and to love and love life as fully as I can. Might sound cheesy but after a cancer diagnosis your whole perspective on what really matters changes. I've a great f*ckit list.

What can I say? Cancer is an extremely complex life event to navigate. It is a rollercoaster of highs and lows. Unpredictable each day. Intense emotions, and real distress. Pain and sadness. Fear and frustration. Yet its paradox is that it can be packed with very special moments of love, support and nurturing. Times of adrenaline-filled highs and incredible experiences. Indeed, it is the hardest challenge I have ever faced, and those closest to me know how I relish a challenge!

Cancer changes lives forever, and now that I'm on board this shuttle, destination unknown, I cannot give enough thanks to the army of people who have boarded with me, helping me from day dot to now. For coaxing me over each hurdle. For celebrating life and each victory with me. In some ways, it has enriched my life, and my personal growth has been immense. As a consequence, I have accomplished so many things I never dreamt that I would ever do …

This year I was told I was cancer free – again. This is now my fourth year since my diagnosis on 21 September 2018, and I am unable to describe to you how happy and relieved I am to have got this far. I know all too well how life can change in a heartbeat.

Cancer, you tried your hardest to tamper and wreak havoc in my life, you tormented my family, my friends, my body, my mind, and my soul. But with the support from you, my dream team of family and friends, and the skill, patience and tenacity of my medical team, plus my own sheer grit, determination, and the 'go nail this' attitude I wear shamelessly on my sleeve, we are barrelling into another year thankfully intact.

Cancer tested us on so many levels. I have fallen off the horse more times than I can count. There have been casualties along the road, and some scars run deep. But I've emerged in the most part, smiling, grateful and proud.

There, I said it. Really proud.

So, as we enter my fifth year of surveillance, I'm scared, but hopeful. And I'm daring, cautiously and optimistically, to plan for a future once again. One where I grow old and grey, with my husband by my side, meet my grandchildren and travel the world. I can hope. Nothing in life is ever a given, but I know I will never take my health for granted. Life has never been so Technicolor, and I'm certainly embracing life, and all that there is on offer.

I promised myself at diagnosis that I would take whatever life throws at me and run with it as best as I can; there have been bumps, potholes, and floods along this path at times, and there were days when I sank deep despite donning a life jacket. Nevertheless, I've managed to fulfil goals and aspirations that the Anisha before cancer could only ever have dreamt of. And if you're reading this and you're facing a hardship, including cancer, or you're some way down the line, know that you, too, can find the courage and strength to keep taking strides along the path laid bare in front of you – step by step, mile by mile, mountain by mountain.

None of us knows what the future holds. I make no resolutions, but instead opt to just go with the flow, taking each day as it comes.

And ultimately, I have an abundance of hope.

Hope is what many of us hold onto tightly, never wanting to let go.

Hope can make the unbearable, bearable.

Hope that we can be cured.

Hope that cancer won't return, or spread further.

Hope that we have more time – more hours, days, months and years with loved ones.

Hope that we can get through treatment, with minimal insult.

Hope that we can drive cancer awareness, break taboos, quash the stigmas and health barriers that surround health-seeking behaviours.

Hope for health equality.

Hope that health professionals listen, do the necessary tests, and diagnose patients early, because we know that early diagnosis saves lives.

Hope that we can advocate for ourselves too.

Hope that further treatments and advances will be made through cancer research to reach a vision of a world where nobody needs die of cancer.

Hope, with a dose of self-advocacy, is what carried me through treatment, clinging on for better days amidst the most difficult ones.

Hope that surgery would be successful, that chemotherapy would mop up any wandering cancer cells.

And hope that I would be cancer-free, to see my children grow up and meet milestones.

I also have a more personal hope – that I can make a difference. Through health promotion, by raising awareness, and through health education in the hope to prevent disease, and by helping others steer their way through their own cancer experiences. I sincerely hope that this book has made a small, positive difference to you whether you have an association with cancer or not.

I hope there was something in here for everyone.

My intention in writing this book was for it to be a companion to those individuals afflicted by this disease, resulting in you feeling less alone and more empowered. More seen. More held. I hope, above all, this book has given you hope of your own, and the tools and information to take the next steps. Hope that you can move forward through a diagnosis of cancer, and come to live well with or after cancer, thriving and surviving. And most importantly, hope that anything is possible in the face of adversity. With the right mindset and support, so much is possible within the new normal. I'm wishing you all the best for treatment and beyond.

To those loved ones around you, I hope this book gives you an insight into the world of cancer, especially bowel cancer, and provides an aid to you.

And to those who have just chosen to read this book of your own accord and who are not directly afflicted by this disease, I hope it has been an education, and it has given you an insight into the world of colorectal cancer, as well as a realistic account of life after a diagnosis.

Remember that life is fragile, a precious commodity, and should never be taken for granted. Advocate for yourself, know your normal, and seek help if you're worried or unsure.

We have only one body, so try to take care of it.

23

Postscript

There is no doubt cancer remains a devastating diagnosis. The cancer journey can be a dark and perilous path of hidden obstacles and trip hazards from which few emerge unscathed. But thanks to scientific advancements and the unwavering dedication of the medical and pharmaceutical communities, its twists and turns are becoming more easily negotiable, journey times extended, and the forward views ever clearer.

None of us is a deliberate explorer of the uncharted territories at journey's end. The first steps on foreign shores need treading carefully, tentatively, until we can stride with poise and purpose and reflect on the distances travelled.

As Einstein theorized, time is related to matter. And what matters most is that whatever time we each have we use wisely, fritter little, and live each day in the best way that we can. Life, after all, is for living.

So what are you waiting for?

Go for it.

The possibilities are infinite.

A ∞

Appendix

Low-residue diet

Why follow a low-fibre/low-residue diet (LRD)?

A low-fibre/low-residue diet is recommended when people need to avoid foods that may irritate an inflamed bowel (such as with Crohn's disease or ulcerative colitis, or an episode of diverticulitis) or if the bowel is narrowed in parts and at risk of obstruction. People are also advised to follow a low-residue diet a few days prior to a colonoscopy to aid preparation of the bowel or following bowel surgery.

What is a low-fibre/low-residue diet?

A low-fibre/low-residue diet is made up of foods that are easily digested and absorbed leaving a minimal residue in the bowel. 'Residue' is essentially undigested food.

The low-residue diet limits dietary fibre to less than 10–15 g per day and restricts other foods that could stimulate bowel activity, which I know feels counter-intuitive with the advice given earlier in the book. However, the aim of a LRD is to decrease the size and frequency of bowel movements, reduce diarrhoea, bloating, excess wind and stomach cramps.

Unsurprisingly, some people find themselves constipated so may need medication to help whilst on this diet, till a point is reached where you are able to reintroduce some fibre.

What can I eat?

Grains

- White breads and plain crackers (unseeded)
- Cooked cereals, like farina, cream of wheat, and grits
- Cold cereals, like puffed rice and corn flakes
- White rice, noodles, and refined pasta

Fruits and vegetables

- Peel the skin and discard any seeds from the fruit and vegetables as these are full of fibre

303

- Well-cooked fresh vegetables or canned vegetables without seeds, like asparagus tips, beetroot, green beans, carrots, mushrooms, spinach, squash, and pumpkin
- Avocado
- Cooked potatoes without skin
- Tomato sauce (no seeds)
- Ripe bananas
- Melon: soft cantaloupe, honeydew
- Tinned or cooked peeled fruits without seeds, for example, apple sauce or canned pears

Drinks

- Decaffeinated drinks including coffee and teas as caffeine can upset your stomach and increase transit through the gut
- Milk (unless lactose intolerant)
- Smooth juices made without seeds or pulp
- Strained vegetable juices

What can't I eat?

You should avoid all high-fibre sources of food. These include:

- Seeds and nuts (including any in breads, jam, cheese etc)
- Whole-grain products (brown), including breads, cereals, crackers, pasta, rice, and kasha
- Raw fruit and most vegetables
- Dried fruits, such as prunes, berries, raisins, figs, and pineapple
- Certain cooked vegetables, including peas, broccoli, winter squash, Brussels sprouts, cabbage, corn (and cornbread), onions, cauliflower, potatoes with skin, and baked beans
- Pulses and tofu
- Tough meats with gristle, and smoked or cured deli meats
- Crunchy peanut butter, jam, marmalade, and preserves
- Pickles, olives, relish, sauerkraut, and horseradish
- Popcorn
- Fruit juices with 'bits' or seeds, prune juice

How long do I need to follow this diet for?

This diet is usually temporary but can sometimes be longer term depending on your condition and symptoms. Your doctor may recommend this diet for a little while when you have a flare-up – an inflamed bowel – or after surgery to help with recovery.

It is worth liaising with a dietitian to discuss how to follow this diet and how to reintroduce foods with more fibre.

If you do not get on with a particular food, it is fine to omit it, but don't give up hope if it used to be a favourite. Once the gut has settled further, it may be worth trying again.

The aim is to find a level of fibre intake that you can manage. Remember to increase your fluid intake as you increase your fibre.

Tips for the reintroduction of fibre/residue foods

Your dietitian or doctor will guide you on how and when to reintroduce fibre/residue into your diet.

From my experience of a low-residue diet after bowel surgery and a stoma, the key to reintroduction was to reintroduce fibre foods SLOWLY, keeping a note of what foods are introduced and what symptoms you experience following ingestion.

Limit foods that you have not been able to manage previously that cause symptoms of discomfort. Don't give up hope, as you could try reintroducing them in a few months' time. Different people can tolerate different levels of fibre intake and residue.

Whilst increasing fibre in your diet, it is important to increase your fluid intake simultaneously. Aim for 8–10 cups of fluid a day.

When introducing new foods, include one at a time, in small amounts (one third of your normal portion).

Ideas for reintroduction

- Try replacing white bread with wholemeal bread.
- Try a higher fibre breakfast cereal such as Weetabix, Shredded Wheat or Bran Flakes.
- Try fruit and vegetables from the 'avoid' list (but continue to avoid dried fruit).
- Five portions of fruit and vegetables (not including potatoes) are recommended in the long term for a healthy diet.

- Try eating the skins on fruit and vegetables such as apples, pears or potatoes.
- If you are still symptom free, try including any of the other foods from the original 'avoid' list, including dried fruit.

If you are struggling, please do ask for help from your specialist nurse or dietitian.

Sleep hygiene

Sleep hygiene is so important to ensuring a good night's sleep. It encompasses a variety of different practices to increase the quality of sleep and therefore improve our wellbeing in the day. It is often an element of wellbeing that is disturbed the most not only for patients but also for loved ones around them, due to the emotional overwhelm and sometimes due to treatment itself.

What people sometimes don't realize is how you plan activity through your day can affect your sleep at night. With this in mind, the tips below take you through the day to ensure that you have a degree of routine and sleep hygiene, to try to achieve a better night's sleep.

- Wake up at the same time each day (and go to bed at a similar time each day).
- Get out in the fresh air and sunlight, which helps maintain a healthy sleep – wake cycle.
- Take regular exercise
- Use the bed for sleep, sickness or sex – avoid using it to watch TV or work in.
- Keep a journal, so any worries of the day or job lists can be written into the journal for safe keeping till the next day. This can help alleviate worry as you drift off to sleep.
- Create a restful bedroom environment:
  o Ensure the room is dark (consider blackout blinds or thick curtains)
  o Use ears plugs, eye masks or a spacemask
  o Keep the room at a comfortable temperature.

- If you are not asleep within 20 minutes, leave your bed and trying reading with a dim light. Try again when you feel sleepy.
- Try a warm bath, relaxing activities in the two hours leading up to bedtime. Mindfulness – try the Headspace or Calm app or meditation or gentle yoga or breathing exercises.

Things to avoid

- Caffeine after 2 p.m. (coffee, tea, chocolate, caffeinated drinks).
- Alcohol in the evening or using it to get to sleep – this disturbs the sleep cycle and is a depressant in itself.
- Smoking in the evening as nicotine is a stimulant.
- Exercise within four hours of your bedtime.
- Too many naps – although napping is a normal part of recovery and in treatment, try to avoid naps longer than 30 minutes.
- Getting frustrated with yourself if you cannot get to sleep, which will awaken your mind even further.
- Going to bed too full or too hungry.

If you still cannot sleep despite taking these measures, please discuss this with your doctor.

Looking after our gut microbiome (GM) – dietary advice

In addition to lifestyle measures to help improve your gut microbiome (sleep, exercise, self-care and stress reduction, etc), there are a number of dietary changes that can help promote a healthy GM.

- Reduce refined sugar. Gut-friendly alternatives for the sweet tooth include honey, dark chocolate, mango, apples, berries and sweet potato.
- Reduce processed food.
- Prebiotics and probiotics – see table below. Eating a balance of these can ensure your gut microbiome is healthily maintained.
- Eat a rainbow of plant-based foods and aim for at least 30 different colourful fruits and vegetables a week. This can increase the number of beneficial bacteria and also act as a fibre source, however, it does not diversify the GM.

- Only take antibiotics if absolutely necessary as they can wipe out your natural GM.
- Reduce red meat: several studies have shown healthier GMs in vegetarians.
- Reduce alcohol consumption which can affect the GM.

Prebiotics: Foods that are a source of fibre for the live bacteria resulting in an increase in the number of bacteria	Probiotics: Foods that are teeming with live beneficial bacteria, that also diversify the GM
Leeks and onions	Fermented foods: sauerkraut, kimchi, kombucha, kefir, unpasteurized pickles
Garlic	Sauerkraut
Jerusalem artichokes	Miso
Berries	Live yoghurts
Nuts and seeds	Sourdough bread
Legumes, pulses and lentils	Kvass (Eastern European fermented cereal drink)
Asparagus	Natto (Japanese fermented soybean product)
Bananas	Dhokla (Indian fermented savoury cake)
Green tea extract	Cheese: Edam, Gouda, cottage cheese, Swiss, Provolone, Gruyere
Wholegrains	
Apples	
Root vegetables	
Bananas	

If your diet is varied, there is rarely a need for food supplementation of these bacteria. However, as I mentioned, I have taken courses of probiotics, especially in the early years post cancer treatment, which provided benefit to my gut. If you choose to do this, seek advice from your doctor first.

If you choose to take food supplements, be aware that you need to be eating a good dose of prebiotics from dietary fibrous sources for the probiotics to work as they rely on prebiotics as their food source. Taking probiotics alone will not be beneficial.

Secondly, the quality between supplements available varies hugely and many don't have any proven efficacy. All supplements have varying concentrations of live bacteria and different types of bacteria, most probiotics need to be refrigerated and kept out of humidity to ensure the organisms are not killed off and inactivated.

There are also a small number of people whose symptoms may worsen and who should not take these supplements (for example those with small intestinal bacterial overgrowth spoken about earlier in the book), so as I mention, seek advice if unsure.

Useful resources

Useful resources and general contacts for further support

General resources A–Z

Age UK ageuk.org.uk – gives health support, care and help specifically for older people.

ALIKE www.alike.org.uk – a charity providing connection via a peer support platform sharing lived experiences.

American Cancer Society www.cancer.org

American Society of Clinical Oncology www.asco.org

Beating Bowel Cancer www.beatingbowelcancer.org

Bowel Cancer UK www.bowelcanceruk.org.uk

Bowel Research UK www.bowelresearchuk.org

Bladder and Bowel Community bladderandbowel.org – an organization providing support and products for people with bladder and bowel control problems.

British Acupuncture Council www.acupuncture.org.uk

British Dietetic Association bda.uk.com – find a dietician in your area.

Cancer Care Map www.cancercaremap.org – helps you locate any local service you may require in the UK.

Cancer Research UK cancerresearchuk.org – information and advice for people affected by cancer.

Cancer Support UK cancersupportuk.org – provides practical and emotional support to people living with cancer, both during and after treatment.

Caring Bridge www.caringbridge.org

Chartered Society of Physiotherapy csp.org.uk

Citizens Advice citizensadvice.org.uk – free, confidential advice on work, finances and housing.

Colon Cancer Coalition (US) www.coloncancercoalition.org

Colon Cancer Foundation (US) www.coloncancerfoundation.org

Colorectal Cancer Alliance (US) www.ccalliance.org

Colon Club (US) www.colonclub.com – supporting those diagnosed under 45 years.

Colostomy Association (for people with a colostomy) colostomy-association.org.uk

Colostomy UK colostomyuk.org

Crohn's and Colitis https://crohnsandcolitis.org.uk

Dietician UK www.dieticianuk.co.uk

Disability Rights UK disabilityrightsuk.org

Dying Matters www.dyingmatters.org

Fighting Colorectal Cancer (US) www.fightingcolorectalcancer.org

GirlsvsCancer www.girlsvscancer.co.uk

GUTS UK www.gutscharity.org.uk

IA (ileostomy and internal pouch) support group iasupport.org

Institute of Cancer Research www.cancerresearchuk.org

Look Good, Feel Better www.lookgoodfeelbetter.co.uk

Live Through This www.livethroughthis.co.uk – the UK's only LGBTQ+ cancer charity.

Macmillan Cancer Support macmillan.org.uk – provides support and information on cancer, money, benefits and work.

Maggie's maggiescentres.org – shares free practical, emotional and social support to people with cancer and their family and friends. Maggie's has centres at some NHS hospitals as well as an online centre.

Marie Curie www.mariecurie.org.uk

Memorial Sloan Kettering Cancer Centre www.mskcc.org

Mission Remission www.mission-remission.com

Mummy's Star www.mummysstar.org

nidirect.gov.uk – government website for Northern Ireland citizens. Includes information on help with health costs.

National Cancer Institute (National Institute of Health) (US) www.cancer.gov – gives information on cancer and treatments.

National Institute for Health and Care Excellence (NICE) www.nice.org.uk

NHS nhs.uk – provides health and lifestyle information, including general information about diet, physical activity, sleep problems, fatigue and emotional support.

NHS Live Well www.nhs.uk/live-well

Patient UK www.patient.co.uk

Pelvic Radiation Disease Association pride.org.uk – support for the effects of radiotherapy

Penny Brohn UK www.pennybrohn.org.uk – helps people live well with cancer by offering a range of services, including wellbeing courses and complementary therapies.

Sex with cancer www.sexwithcancer.com

Sexual Advice Association sexualadviceassociation.co.uk – offers information on sex and intimacy, including information for people with cancer.

Shine Cancer Support shinecancersupport.org – a charity that exclusively supports adults in their 20s, 30s and 40s who have had a cancer diagnosis.

Stand Up to Cancer www.standuptocancer.org.uk

St Marks https://www.stmarkshospital.nhs.uk/patients-visitors/patient-information-leaflets/ – the National Bowel Hospital.

Teens Unite www.teensunite.org – a charity supporting teens and young adults affected by cancer.

The Royal Surrey NHS Foundation Trust https://www.royalsurrey.nhs.uk/useful-links-and-resources-/ – useful patient links.

Trekstock www.trekstock.com – cancer charity for young adults.

You, Me and the Big C www.bbc.co.uk/youmebigc – podcast.

Books

The Bowel Cancer Recovery Toolkit by Sarah Russell (Hammersmith Press Ltd, 2019)

The Cancer Survivor's Companion by Dr Frances Goodhart and Lucy Atkins (Piatkus, 2013)

How to Live When You Could Be Dead by Dame Deborah James (Ebury, 2022)

The Complete Guide to POI and Early Menopause by Dr Hannah Short and Dr Mandy Leonhardt (Sheldon Press, 2022)

Yoga for Cancer by Vicky Fox (Hammersmith Health Books, 2022)

Resources for parents

Fruitfly Collective www.fruitflycollective.com

Hope Support Services www.hopesupport.org.uk

Little C Club flash cards www.littlecclub.com – I was fortunate to receive these as a gift and they are ideal for those aged 2–10 years.

Macmillan Cancer Support www.macmillan.org.uk – there is a guide called 'Talking to children and teenagers when an adult has cancer'.

Rip Rap www.riprap.org.uk – support for teenagers.

UK Trauma Council www.uktraumacouncil.org

Young Minds www.youngminds.org.uk

Winston's Wish www.winstonswish.org.uk

The Fountain Centre has a recommended list of books for parents and children www.fountaincentre.org/general-family-and-child-support.html

Resources for carers

All the main cancer charities also have pages supporting carers.

Carers UK www.carersuk.org

Carers Trust www.carers.org

Carers First www.carersfirst.org.uk

Cancer-friendly gifts

Cancer Research UK https://shop.cancerresearchuk.org/cancer-care

The C-List https://www.the-c-list.com

Not Another Bunch of Flowers www.notanotherbunchofflowers.com

Look Good, Feel Better https://shop.lookgoodfeelbetter.co.uk

Beauty Despite Cancer by Jennifer Young www.beautydespitecancer.com

Return to work resources

Working With Cancer:
https://workingwithcancer.co.uk/best-practice-guides

https://workingwithcancer.co.uk/job-seekers/career-coaching-workbook/

https://workingwithcancer.co.uk/content/files/Your-rights-at-work.pdf

Maggies:

https://www.maggies.org/cancer-support/managing-practically/work-and-cancer/

https://www.maggies.org/cancer-support/managing-practically/driving-and-cancer/

Macmillan:

https://www.macmillan.org.uk/cancer-information-and-support/stories-and-media/booklets/work-and-cancer

https://www.macmillan.org.uk/cancer-information-and-support/impacts-of-cancer/self-employment-and-cancer

https://www.macmillan.org.uk/cancer-information-and-support/get-help/financial-and-work

Try also:

Access to work scheme https://www.gov.uk/access-to-work/after-you-apply

In the US, this website may also help with financial support https://www.cancer.net/navigating-cancer-care/financial-considerations/financial-resources

https://www.cancer.gov/about-cancer/managing-care/track-care-costs

ACAS acas.org.uk – provides free information and advice on problems in the workplace and employment law.

Department for Work and Pensions www.dwp.gov.uk – for information on benefits, work and disability.

TUC: Trades Union Congress www.worksmart.org.uk – information regarding employment and disability rights.

Mental health resources

Explore the websites of the following organizations (see A–Z in general resources above for websites):

American Cancer Society

Cancer Research UK

Macmillan

MIND and YOUNG MINDS

Trekstock
Shine Cancer Support – for those in their 20s, 30s and 40s
For mindfulness and relaxation try:
Stress No More www.stressnomore.co.uk
Headspace www.headspace.com
Calm www.calm.com
Breathing Tree www.breathingtree.co.uk
Breathpod www.breathpod.com

Survivorship

The American Society for Cancer produces the following document: https://www.asco.org/sites/new-www.asco.org/files/content-files/practice-and-guidelines/documents/colorectal-cancer-treatment-summary-and-survivorship-care-plan.docx

Exercise

NHS Couch to 5k
    5K Your Way https://5kyourway.org
    Trekstock
    Move Against Cancer www.movecharity.org
    CancerFit www.cancerfit.me
    Fighting Fit for Cancer https://www.ffit4c.com

LARS

Bowel Cancer UK have a leaflet called 'Regaining bowel control' with useful nuggets and advice. You can download it from their website and it has lots of useful information.

Try also: https://livingwithlars.com/management-tips/ – this website has been set up by members of the Facebook team in a bid to help individuals with problematic symptoms.

Menopause and fertility

COTS: Childlessness Overcome Through Surrogacy www.surrogacy.org.uk

Adoption UK www.adoptionuk.org

The Daisy Network www.daisynetwork.org.uk – for women dealing with premature menopause (premature ovarian insufficiency).

Balance https://www.balance-menopause.com – a menopause library.

The Menopause Charity www.themenopausecharity.org

Menopause Care https://menopausecare.co.uk

Menopause and Me www.menopauseandme.co.uk

LGBTQ+

The National LGBT cancer network is a fabulous website offering support as well as a CRC toolkit: https://colorectalcancer.cancer-network.org/

They also offer a Facebook group for those affected by CRC https://www.facebook.com/groups/1448440288756634/?ref=group_header

Live Through This www.livethroughthis.co.uk – for those with cancer in the LGBTQ community.

In the US, the LGBTQ+ cancer project is also available with support: https://www.lgbtcancer.org

Genetic support groups

Lynch Syndrome UK https://www.lynch-syndrome-uk.org/

Lynch Syndrome Ireland https://lynchsyndromeireland.com/

Genetic Alliance UK also lists other polyp patient support groups such as for FAP: https://geneticalliance.org.uk/member/fap-gene-support-group/

Fight Lynch (US) www.fightlynch.org

Ethnic minority support resources

Black Women Rising www.blackwomenrisinguk.org – support group for people of colour who have been diagnosed with cancer. They are here to support, educate and break down taboos and stigma within cultural beliefs regarding cancer and they connect sharing each other's experiences. I have done a podcast for them too.

Asian Women Cancer Group https://www.asianwomencancergroup. co.uk

Bereavement support

This can be obtained from the hospice if your loved one was a patient there. Other organizations include:
Cruse Bereavement Care (UK) www.cruse.org.uk/
The Loss Foundation https://www.thelossfoundation.org
Facebook support groups include:
Living with Stage 4
Living with Low Anterior Resection Syndrome
Bowel Cancer Support Group

Travel insurance

A question I'm often asked about is regarding travel insurance, as unfortunately having cancer can impact this. Here are a few recommendations:
Free Spirit Travel Insurance www.freespirittravelinsurance.com
Freedom Insurance www.freedominsure.co.uk
Insurancewith www.insurancewith.com
Insurance Choice www.insurancechoice.co.uk
Insure Cancer www.insurecancer.com
J D Travel Insurance www.jdtravelinsurance.co.uk
Orbis Insurance www.orbisinsurance.co.uk

End of life

Cancer Research have the following resource: https://www.cancerresearchuk.org/about-cancer/coping/dying-with-cancer/last-few-weeks-and-days/final-days

Glossary

Adjuvant chemotherapy   Given after surgery, the goal of chemotherapy is to kill cancer cells that may have been left behind at surgery as they were too small to see, as well as cancer cells that may have escaped to other parts of the body, that are undetectable on scans at the time.

Anastomosis   This is a surgical connection or joint between two structures, for example when the bowel cancer is removed, the two remaining ends of the bowel are sewn or stapled back together.

Anterior resection   An operation performed for rectal cancers where part of the rectum and colon are removed and then the bowel ends eventually rejoined.

CEA (carcinoembryonic antigen)   A protein that is produced by some types of cancers such as CRC. It can be used to monitor treatment and surveillance.

HIPEC (hyperthermic intraperitoneal chemotherapy)   A type of therapy used in advanced abdominal cancers using both surgery and warmed chemotherapy agents as a method of treatment.

Ileostomy   Small bowel is diverted to the surface of the skin, opening up in the tummy wall. A bag is placed over the opening to collect the stool.

Immunotherapy   A type of treatment that uses your immune system to destroy cancer cells.

Laparoscopic   Keyhole surgery.

Lymph node   There are hundreds of small bean shaped structures around the body that form part of the immune system. If cancer spreads, it can spread to the lymph nodes via the lymphatic system.

Neoadjuvant chemoradiotherapy   Chemotherapy and radiotherapy given before surgery with the goal of reducing tumour size so it is more amenable to surgery, as well as potentially treating undetected micrometastasis.

Oncologist   A specialist doctor who uses cancer treatments (chemotherapy, radiotherapy, immunotherapy and a range of other treatments) to manage patients with cancer.

Palliative care   Specialized medical care and support for the patient and their family, via a multidisciplinary approach for those with a serious medical illness or a life-limiting condition. The aim is to improve quality of life.

Pathologist   A specialist doctor who studies the biopsies and tissue samples taken for cancer cells sent from procedures.

PIPAC (pressurized intraperitoneal aerosol chemotherapy)   A procedure used in advanced abdominal cancer involving administering chemotherapy through the abdominal cavity in aerosol form.

Portacath   A small medical device which sits under your skin on your chest wall, attached to a catheter sitting in a large vein close to your heart. It is used to draw blood and give treatments (including blood, chemotherapy, fluids, antibiotics or blood transfusions).

Pelvic exenteration   An operation to remove multiple organs in the pelvis affected by cancer.

Peritoneum   A thin layer of tissue that lines the inside of the abdomen.

PICC line   Peripherally inserted central catheter – a long cannula inserted into the vein in the upper arm to administer treatment.

Radiologist   A specialist who uses imaging to diagnose, manage and treat patients.

Stoma   An opening in the body.

Total mesenteric excision   A specific surgical technique used in the management of rectal cancers in which the bowel containing the cancer is entirely removed along with the surrounding fat and lymph nodes to reduce the chance of local recurrence.

Contributors

Professor Timothy Rockall (Consultant Colorectal Surgeon) is a Consultant Surgeon at the Royal Surrey County Hospital Guildford and Professor of Surgery at the University of Surrey and Director of the Minimal Access Therapy Training Unit (MATTU) in Guildford. He specializes in laparoscopic gastrointestinal surgery and has a particular interest and expertise in the practice and teaching of laparoscopic colorectal surgery. He was previously Senior Lecturer at Imperial College, London in the department of Surgical Technology and Oncology, and Honorary Consultant at St Mary's Hospital London. He is Past President of the Association of Laparoscopic Surgeons of Great Britain and Ireland, and is currently a Council member of the Royal College of Surgeons of England (RCSE).

Dr Alexandra Stewart is a Consultant Clinical Oncologist specializing in gynaecological and lower GI cancers. She has a specialist interest in dynamic optimization of radiotherapy particularly using adaptive external beam radiotherapy and brachytherapy. She qualified in 1997 and trained at Charing Cross and the Royal Marsden Hospitals with a Fellowship at Harvard University in Boston. She works at the Royal Surrey County Hospital in Guildford, leading the brachytherapy service. She participates in committees for the BIR, RCR and ESTRO, focusing on research, education and quality improvement in radiotherapy.

Mrs Angela Bates is a Clinical Colorectal Nurse Specialist working at Royal Surrey Foundation NHS Trust, Guildford. She has over 25 years' experience specializing in colorectal cancer, working both in the surgical and oncological setting, and has a Masters in advanced practice in cancer care. She has also previously held the position of enhanced recovery nursing champion with the Kent, Surrey & Sussex Academic Health Science Network and facilitated the implementation of the Enhanced Recovery programme within her Trust and the acute hospitals in the South East.

Dr Katie Snape is a Consultant in Cancer Genetics and a Reader in Clinical Genomics. Katie has a PhD in molecular genetics from the Institute of Cancer Research and a Postgraduate Certificate in

Healthcare and Biomedical Education. Katie is a Fellow of the Higher Education Academy and Secretary of the UK Cancer Genetics Group. Katie's clinical and academic focus is on trying to innovate and improve healthcare systems and pathways to improve the clinical care of people with increased genetic risk of developing cancer.

Dr Gareth Sadler is a Consultant Gastroenterologist at St George's Hospital, Tooting, London. He has previously held the posts of Endoscopy Training Lead and Director of the South West London Bowel Cancer Screening Programme, and is currently the Director of Endoscopy at St George's Hospital. He is a JAG-accredited bowel cancer screening colonoscopist, an assessor of aspirant endoscopists to the bowel cancer screening programme, and a member of the national bowel cancer screening programme's accreditation panel. He is a core faculty member and lead of JAG-accredited endoscopy courses at St George's Hospital, a national endoscopy training centre. He co-leads the advanced colonoscopy resection service at St George's Hospital with Dr Kesavan Kandiah, treating advanced colonic polyps and very early bowel cancer using advanced endoscopy techniques.

He is married to **Dr Anisha Patel**, and in addition to his professional expertise, he has first-hand experience of being a close relative of a patient with bowel cancer!

Danielle Freeth is a psychotherapist and clinical supervisor working in private practice and as the Psychological Lead at the Fountain Centre, a small independent cancer charity based within an NHS Trust. Danielle has vast experience of working with adults, couples, children and families.

Index

abdominal cavity, spread of cancer to, 116
abdomino-perineal resection, 60
ablative therapies, 111–12, 115
acupuncture, 105, 185
adjuvant therapy, 79, 318
adoption, 190
advanced colorectal cancer, 32, 109–19, 193–4
aftermath of cancer, xxiii, 139–53, 272–84, 297–300
  age as a risk factor, 15, 22–3
alcohol, 14, 176, 185
alternative therapies, 44
anaemia, xxii, 27, 97
anal canal, 3, 60, 177
anal sphincter muscle exercises, 172–3
anger, 99–100, 201–2
angiogenesis inhibitors, 124–5
anniversaries, 278
anterior resection surgery, *58*, *59*, 318
anxiety, xxv, 29, 211–13, 215–20, 222
  fear of recurrence, 191–3, 195–9, 263
appetite loss, 83, 95–6
aspirin, 21

bacteria in the gut, 11, 21
balance exercises, 156
bereavement charities, 317
bile acid malabsorption (BAM), 170–1
Black Women Rising, 288, 316–17
bladder dysfunction, 88–9
blood in stools, xxii–xxiii, 6
blood tests, 27, 81, 195
bowel, layers, *56*
bowel cancer *see* colorectal cancer (CRC)
bowel cancer screening (BCS), 20, 21, 292–6
bowel control clinics, 177–8
bowel habits, 4, 6, 176, 193
bowel obstruction, 63–5
bowel urgency, xxii, 7
BRAF genes, 124, 125–6
brain fog, 97–9
breastfeeding, 291

breathing exercises, 234–5
Bristol Stool Chart, 4–5
bruising, 97

campaigning, 284
Cancer Card, 276–8
cancer community, 281–2
capecitabine, side effects, 81–4, 106–7
carers, 247–9, 313
CEA (carcinoembryonic antigen), 28, 195, 318
chemo-radiotherapy, xxv–xxvi, 80–4
chemotherapy, 92–3, 127–9, 133–4
  drug-free week, 129–30, 257–8
  exercise during, 159
  and pregnancy, 291
  resistance to, 125
  side effects, 94–108, 160–6, 188
children, 35–40, 46, 254–60, 313
claustrophobia, 29, 222
clinical cancer nurse specialists (CNSs), 48–9, 52–3
cognitive behavioural therapy (CBT), 152–3, 185, 222, 237–8 *see also* trauma-based CBT
cold sensitivity, side effect of oxaliplatin, 103–6
cologuard test, 25
colon, 3, *4*, 58
colonoscopy, xxiii–xxiv, 6, 25–7, 195
colorectal cancer (CRC)
  definition, 6
  progression, *56*
  symptoms, xxii–xxiii, 6–7
colorectal specialist nurses, 169, 176
colostomy, 73, *73*, 78 *see also* stoma
communication, 228
compassion-focused therapy (CFT), 226–7
constipation, xxii, 82
contrast dye, 28
cooking methods, 10
counselling, 50, 175, 209, 211, 236–7
  for children, 39, 257
  for partners, 246